NURSING PHOTOBOOK™

Implementing Urologic Procedures

NURSING83 BOOKS™
SPRINGHOUSE CORPORATION
SPRINGHOUSE, PENNSYLVANIA

***NURSING83* BOOKS**™

NURSING PHOTOBOOK™ SERIES
Providing Respiratory Care
Managing I.V. Therapy
Dealing with Emergencies
Giving Medications
Assessing Your Patients
Using Monitors
Providing Early Mobility
Giving Cardiac Care
Performing GI Procedures
Implementing Urologic Procedures
Controlling Infection
Ensuring Intensive Care
Coping with Neurologic Disorders
Caring for Surgical Patients
Working with Orthopedic Patients
Nursing Pediatric Patients
Helping Geriatric Patients
Attending Ob/Gyn Patients
Aiding Ambulatory Patients
Carrying Out Special Procedures

NURSING SKILLBOOK® SERIES
Dealing with Death and Dying
Reading EKGs Correctly
Managing Diabetics Properly
Assessing Vital Functions Accurately
Helping Cancer Patients Effectively
Giving Cardiovascular Drugs Safely
Giving Emergency Care Competently
Monitoring Fluid and Electrolytes Precisely
Documenting Patient Care Responsibly
Combatting Cardiovascular Diseases Skillfully
Coping with Neurologic Problems Proficiently
Nursing Critically Ill Patients Confidently
Using Crisis Intervention Wisely

NURSE'S REFERENCE LIBRARY®
Diseases
Diagnostics
Drugs
Assessment
Procedures
Definitions

***Nursing83* DRUG HANDBOOK™**

NURSING PHOTOBOOK™ Series

PUBLISHER
Eugene W. Jackson

EDITORIAL DIRECTOR
Jean Robinson

CLINICAL DIRECTOR
Barbara McVan, RN

ART DIRECTOR
Lisa A. Gilde

**Springhouse Corporation
Book Division**

DIRECTOR
Timothy B. King

DIRECTOR, RESEARCH
Elizabeth O'Brien

VICE-PRESIDENT, PRODUCTION AND
PURCHASING
Bacil Guiley

Staff for this volume

BOOK EDITOR
Richard Samuel West

CLINICAL EDITOR
Kathleen Soneki Waring, RN

ASSOCIATE EDITOR
Patricia K. Lawson

PHOTOGRAPHER
Paul A. Cohen

ASSOCIATE DESIGNERS
Linda Jovinelly Franklin
Carol Stickles

DESIGN ASSISTANT
Darcy Moore Feralio

ASSOCIATE PHOTOGRAPHER
Thomas Staudenmayer

EDITORIAL/GRAPHIC COORDINATOR
Doreen K. Stowers

CLINICAL/GRAPHIC COORDINATOR
Evelyn M. James

COPY EDITOR
Eric R. Rinehimer

EDITORIAL STAFF ASSISTANT
Cynthia A. O'Connell

PHOTOGRAPHY ASSISTANT
Frank Margeson

ART PRODUCTION MANAGER
Robert Perry

ARTISTS
Diane Fox   Bob Walsh
Sandra Simms   Joan Walsh
Louise Stamper   Ron Yablon

TYPOGRAPHY MANAGER
David C. Kosten

TYPOGRAPHY ASSISTANTS
Janice Auch Haber
Ethel Halle
Diane Paluba
Nancy Wirs

PRODUCTION MANAGERS
Robert L. Dean, Jr.
Kathy Murphy

ASSISTANT PRODUCTION MANAGER
Deborah C. Meiris

PRODUCTION ASSISTANT
Donald G. Knauss

ILLUSTRATORS
Jack Crane   Robert Jackson
John Dougherty   Pat Macht
Jean Gardner   Dennis Schofield
Tom Herbert   Bud Yingling

SERIES GRAPHIC DESIGNER
John C. Isely

COVER PHOTO
Seymour Mednick

**Clinical consultants
for this volume**

Audrey A. Beilman, RN, BSN
Urology Head Nurse
James A. Haley VA Medical Center
Tampa, Fla.

Jean M. Boyle, RN
Urology Nurse
Trenton, N.J.

June L. Stark, RN
Critical Care Instructor
Tufts New England Center Hospital
Boston

Amended reprint, 1983
© 1982, 1981 by Springhouse Corporation, 1111
Bethlehem Pike, Springhouse, PA 19477
All rights reserved. Reproduction in whole or
part by any means whatsoever without written
permission of the publisher is prohibited by law.
Printed in the United States of America.

PB-041083

Library of Congress Cataloging in Publication Data

Main entry under title:

Implementing urologic procedures.

(Nursing81 books) (Nursing Photobook)
Bibliography: p.
Includes index.
1. Urological nursing—Atlases. I. Series.
[DNLM: 1. Urology—Nursing texts.
WY 164 I34]
RC874.7.I48   610.73'69   81-2939
ISBN 0-916730-32-8   AACR2

Contents

Contributors

At the time of original publication, these contributors held the following positions.

Audrey A. Beilman, an adviser for this PHOTOBOOK, is head nurse in the Urology Department, James A. Haley VA Medical Center, Tampa, Florida. She earned a nursing diploma at Mercy Central School of Nursing, Grand Rapids, Michigan, and a BSN degree at the Hampton Institute, Hampton, Virginia. She belongs to the National Honor Society of Nursing.

Jean M. Boyle, an adviser for this PHOTOBOOK, is a urology nurse working in a private practice in Trenton, New Jersey. She earned a nursing diploma at St. Francis Nursing School in Trenton, and has done independent study at Trenton State College and Bucks County (Pa.) Community College.

Marcia Goldstein, head nurse of the Renal-Dialysis Department at Albert Einstein Medical Center (Northern Division), Philadelphia, also is a Certified Hemodialysis Nurse. She earned a nursing diploma at Einstein, and is a member of the American Association of Nephrology Nurses and Technicians, American Association of Critical-Care Nurses, and Southeastern Pa. Critical-Care Nurses.

Diane Kaschak is a transplant nurse clinician at Albert Einstein Medical Center (Northern Division), Philadelphia. She earned a nursing diploma at the School of Nursing, Hospital of the University of Pennsylvania, Philadelphia. She's a member of the National Association of Transplant Coordinators, and the American Association of Nephrology Nurses and Technicians.

Patricia A. McFarland is an enterostomal therapist and ambulatory care staff nurse at the James A. Haley VA Medical Center, Tampa, Florida. She earned a nursing diploma at Stuart Circle Hospital School for Nurses, Richmond, Virginia, and ET certification at Emory University School for Enterostomal Therapy, Atlanta. Ms. McFarland is a member of the Florida Nurses Association, and the International Association for Enterostomal Therapy.

Terry Payton is a urologic nurse clinician at the Boston University Medical Center. He earned an Associate Degree in nursing at Middlesex Community College, Bedford, Massachusetts. He's a member of the Massachusetts Nurses Association, and the American Urological Association, Allied.

Nida L. Quirong is assistant head nurse, hemodialysis unit, and nurse in charge of the CAPD program, Albert Einstein Medical Center (Northern Division), Philadelphia. She earned a nursing diploma at Southwestern University, Cebu City, Philippines, and she belongs to the American Association of Nephrology Nurses and Technicians.

June L. Stark, an adviser for this PHOTOBOOK, is critical-care instructor for staff education at Tufts New England Medical Center Hospital in Boston, where she is also a renal nurse consultant. Ms. Stark earned a nursing diploma at Jackson Memorial Hospital School of Nursing in Miami. She is a member of the American Association of Critical-Care Nurses.

James L. Williams is a urologist's assistant at the University of California Medical Center, San Diego University Hospital. He's a member of the American Urological Association, Allied.

Elizabeth Wright is head nurse of the Urology and Kidney-Transplant Department at Toronto Western Hospital in Toronto. She earned a nursing diploma at Kilmarnock Infirmary, Scotland, and took general training for 3 years and studied midwifery for 1 year in Scotland.

Introduction

No matter where you work, you probably perform some urologic care frequently. From taking a urine specimen to caring for your patient after complicated urinary tract surgery, urologic concerns are part of your day. This PHOTOBOOK examines all major aspects of urologic care, focusing on key steps along the way.

To assess your patient's urinary system, you must know what questions to ask. In our section on patient assessment, we explore questions on a wide variety of topics: your patient's medical history, his allergies, and possible sexual problems—in short, anything that involves his urinary system. You might also have to prepare your patient for one or several diagnostic tests, such as cystography or a computerized tomogram (CT scan). We've profiled how each test is performed and given you information designed to share with your patient.

Performing urethral catheterization isn't difficult, but performing it without introducing harmful bacteria into your patient's urinary tract is. That's why the comprehensive catheterization section in this PHOTOBOOK zeros in on how to perform catheterization procedures *without* infecting your patient. One way you can reduce infection risks is by teaching your patient important self-catheterization techniques. We've devoted over a dozen pages to detailed home care aids on self-catheterization, which you can copy and use to teach your patient.

If the doctor decides surgery's necessary, you may have to manage your patient's preoperative and postoperative care. Vigilance takes top priority in this care. If you know how to detect, for example, electrolyte imbalance or internal hemorrhage, you can catch problems early and prevent them from developing into major complications.

Suppose your patient returns from surgery with an ostomy. You know this surgery will have a major effect on the patient's body image, but do you know how you can put him at ease with himself and make his rehabilitation go smoothly? Our section on caring for the ostomate provides you with some psychologic tools you'll need to guide your patient toward resuming a normal lifestyle.

You'll find that in caring for the patient who requires dialysis or a renal transplant, your biggest challenge is to acquire the knowledge you need. To help you attain this goal, we've packed the section on caring for these patients with useful information, organized in a manner that's easy to follow.

That's the emphasis of IMPLEMENTING UROLOGIC PROCEDURES—presenting valuable information in a logical, useful way. Read this PHOTOBOOK carefully and remember what's in it. We're sure you can take this information and make it work for you.

4 OZ

100 CC

3 OZ

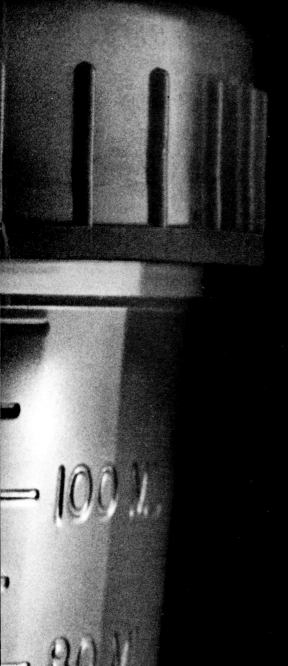

Examining Your Patient's Urinary System

Patient assessment

Patient assessment

You've probably admitted urology patients any number of times. And, as part of the process, you've done a detailed nursing assessment, including questions specific to his condition; done kidney/bladder inspection and palpation; and undertaken patient teaching regarding urine specimens. Sure, you know these tasks well—but do you know them as well as you should? Test your knowledge with these questions:
• What implications does arthritis have in the care and treatment of a urology patient?
• Why must you know whether or not your patient has a respiratory condition?
• How is a cystogram taken and what should the patient know beforehand?
You'll learn the answers to these questions, and much more, in the pages that follow.

Understanding basic anatomy and physiology

You studied urinary tract anatomy and physiology in school. How much do you remember? Use the information that follows to refresh your memory of urologic basics. We've organized our discussion around these four groupings of urinary tract structures: the adrenal glands and kidneys; the ureters; the bladder; and the urethra, prostate gland and reproductive organs.

The adrenal glands and kidneys. Your patient should have two adrenal glands, one capping each kidney. The right adrenal is triangular shaped; the left is more rounded and crescent shaped. Each gland consists of a cortex and a medulla.

The adrenal cortex secretes corticosteroids that control the body's metabolism of fat, protein, and carbohydrates; help the body retain sodium and excrete potassium, which in turn, affects fluid and electrolyte balance; and cause body growth and increase masculine secondary sex characteristics.

The medulla secretes adrenalin and noradrenalin. Adrenalin constricts arterioles in the skin and mucous membranes; relaxes the smooth muscles in the bronchioles of the lungs; raises the blood sugar level; and affects gastric motility and metabolic activity. Noradrenalin maintains vascular constriction and increases the rate and force of cardiac contractions, which, in turn, increases cardiac output and arterial pressure.

The kidneys are positioned between the thoracic and the lumbar regions. They are reddish brown, bean-shaped organs, each about the length and width of an adult's fist, though somewhat thinner. Each kidney contains approximately 1 million nephrons. The nephrons process about 200 quarts of blood daily, accomplishing these four major functions:
• excretion of excess water and nitrogenous waste products of metabolism (chiefly creatine and urea)
• conservation and reabsorption of essential substances in the blood
• regulation of the acid-base balance, volume, and electrolyte concentration of the plasma
• secretion of hormones essential to blood flow and arterial pressure. These

hormones include renin, a potent hypertensive, and erythropoietin, a bone marrow stimulant for the production of red blood cells.

The kidney reabsorbs 99% of the fluids carried in the blood. The remaining 1% becomes urine and is excreted. The waste products are passed out of the kidneys, through the calices and the renal pelvis, to the ureters.

The ureters. Ureters in an adult are about 12″ (30 cm) long, varying in length directly proportional to the height of the individual. Urine travels through the ureters to the bladder.

The bladder. The bladder is an ovoid, hollow, muscular organ about 4″ (10.2 cm) long. It functions as a urine reservoir, usually holding 200 to 300 ml, but with a capacity several times that. When empty, the bladder's located just underneath the symphysis pubis. When full, the bladder rises above the symphysis pubis and can be readily palpated or percussed. Bladder filling stimulates nerve endings that send a message to the brain to urinate. The bladder neck then relaxes, allowing urine to flow from the bladder into and through the urethra to outside the body.

The urethra, prostate gland, and reproductive organs. A female's urethra is a 1″ to 1½″ (2.5 to 3.8 cm) tube that leads directly from the bladder to the perineum, opening anterior to the vagina. As you know, the female urinary tract is distinct and separate from the female reproductive tract.

The male urethra is a 2½″ to 3″ (6.4 to 7.6 cm) tube that travels from the bladder, around the sexual organs, to the head of the penis. The organs near the male urethra include:
• the prostate gland, which lies behind the bladder and helps manufacture ejaculation fluid and acid phosphatase
• the epididymis, which is connected to the top of the testes and stores sperm
• the testes, which are located in the scrotum and produce sperm and testosterone
• the scrotum, which hangs underneath the base of the penis, supporting the testes and regulating their temperature.

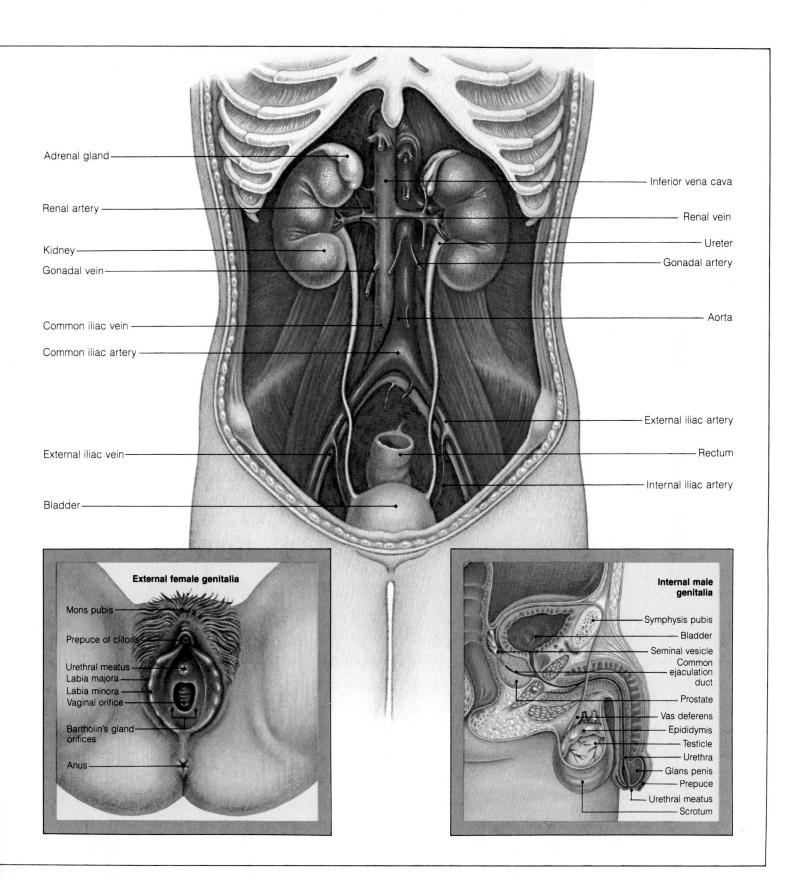

Adrenal gland

Renal artery

Kidney

Gonadal vein

Common iliac vein

Common iliac artery

External iliac vein

Bladder

Inferior vena cava

Renal vein

Ureter

Gonadal artery

Aorta

External iliac artery

Rectum

Internal iliac artery

External female genitalia

Mons pubis

Prepuce of clitoris

Urethral meatus
Labia majora
Labia minora
Vaginal orifice

Bartholin's gland
orifices

Anus

**Internal male
genitalia**

Symphysis pubis
Bladder
Seminal vesicle
Common
ejaculation
duct
Prostate
Vas deferens
Epididymis
Testicle
Urethra
Glans penis
Prepuce
Urethral meatus
Scrotum

Patient assessment

How to compile your patient's medical history

Compiling your patient's medical history is simple but important work. The information you gather will provide you with inside knowledge of your patient's medical problems, past and present. By compiling an accurate history early, you can prevent errors and misunderstandings later. Moreover, the interview provides the perfect opportunity for you to get to know your patient better. Conduct the interview skillfully and you'll establish a good rapport that will last throughout your patient's hospital stay.

Remember, the majority of patients with urologic problems are of an age when they may have a variety of other medical complications. Consequently, be watchful for problems beyond the ones suggested by the admitting diagnosis. That's why the questions you ask during your initial interview must be wide ranging.

Your hospital may use printed forms for this initial interview. If not, base your interview on the guidelines that follow.

Conduct the interview in privacy. Put your patient at ease by being informal and friendly. Don't act rushed. Show interest in the patient as a person. Observe his mental state. If he's confused, depressed, or apprehensive, consider this not only during the interview, but also throughout your care for him. Start here:

• Establish your patient's identity. Ask your patient his name, age, sex, race, nationality, language, religion, marital status, occupation, and referral source.

• Take your patient's vital signs; for example, *record his temperature.* If it's elevated, this may indicate an infection or ureteral obstruction caused by calculi. *Take his blood pressure.* High blood pressure could be a sign of chronic renal disease, renal artery stenosis, adrenal abnormalities, or cardiovascular disease. *Record his pulse.* Note its rate, strength, and regularity. Abnormalities here could indicate cardiac problems. *Weigh the patient.* Has he gained a significant amount of weight recently? This may indicate he's retaining fluid and his kidneys are malfunctioning. But, don't assume weight gain means fluid retention or kidney problems. If your patient's female, find out when her last menstrual period was. It may prove significant.

• Identify the patient's problem by asking him to state his chief complaint. Then, find out if he's experiencing any other discomfort. Include all details of his complaint, and be specific. Ask him when the discomfort began. To probe further, use the list of questions on page 12.

• Record the patient's history. Ask the following questions:

Are you presently taking any drugs? If so, what are they? How much do you take and how often?

Stay alert for possible drug incompatibility, but also learn how various drugs can affect the urinary tract. For example, Valium and other tranquilizers can cause urinary retention by interfering with the bladder's nerve supply and by affecting its ability to contract. Diuretics, which increase urinary excretion of water and sodium, are commonly used to treat hypertension and fluid retention. But, they also deplete the body's potassium content, which can cause dangerous cardiac arrhythmias.

Are you allergic to any drugs? Are you allergic to shellfish? Do you know if you're allergic to iodine or isotope dyes? Do you suffer from asthma or hay fever?

Discover this information to avoid allergic reactions in your patient. For example, if he's allergic to shellfish, that may indicate an allergy to iodine. For such a patient, you won't use any iodine-based dye for X-ray studies. Or, if he's asthmatic, that may indicate heightened physiologic sensitivity, which could cause an allergic reaction to the dye. For such a patient, proceed with caution.

Are you on a special diet; for example, a low-salt diet? Have you been told not to eat foods such as bread or crackers? Have you

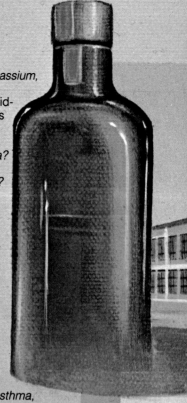

been told to eat foods that are high in potassium, such as bananas?

Such guidelines may be dictated by kidney problems and will affect the patient's fluid and electrolyte levels.

Do you suffer from arthritis or a congenital abnormality, such as spina bifida? Have you ever had hip or spinal surgery? Do you have any partial paralysis? Are you an amputee?

An affirmative answer to any of these questions would contraindicate putting the patient in the lithotomy position for diagnostic procedures or surgery, either because it would be impossible or would cause the patient undue pain.

Have you ever suffered a traumatic spinal-cord injury?

If so, your patient may have a neurogenic bladder disorder. Such a disorder manifests itself as a spastic bladder with persistent incontinence or as an atonic bladder with retention or overflow incontinence.

Do you have (or have you ever had) asthma, bronchitis, pneumonia, or chronic obstructive pulmonary disease? Do you smoke? If so, how much?

Positive answers to these questions call for special care during and immediately after surgery. As you know, the stress of surgery can severely aggravate an asthmatic condition. In addition, the introduction of an endotracheal tube during surgery can cause bronchospasms, impairing respirations. By adjusting your patient's pre- and postop respiratory therapy to accommodate these respiratory problems, you can help prevent pneumonia and postop atelectasis.

Are you a diabetic?

If so, your patient's diabetes may be contributing to or causing his renal problems. Diabetes can also affect postsurgical wound healing. Check the patient's urine-test results for his glucose level. Remember, a diabetic patient's probably on a special diet. The doctor will have to accommodate that diet if he wants to control what the patient eats.

Do you have high blood pressure?

This may be caused by difficulties in urinating, or a malfunctioning kidney.

Can you control your bowel movements? Do you take a laxative regularly?

The state of your patient's bowel can affect his urinary tract. For example, chronic constipation can affect bladder function and cause dehydration. You must determine whether or not your patient's bowels move naturally before you can give him effective postop care.

• Record his family's medical history to determine your patient's total medical picture. Include the ages of the patient's immediate family, plus data on their current health. Also, record the cause of death of any immediate family member.

• Record the patient's personal and social history. For example, ask about his job (how active and demanding it is); his drinking habits (how much alcohol, tea, and coffee he drinks); and his leisure-time activities (how much exercise he gets).

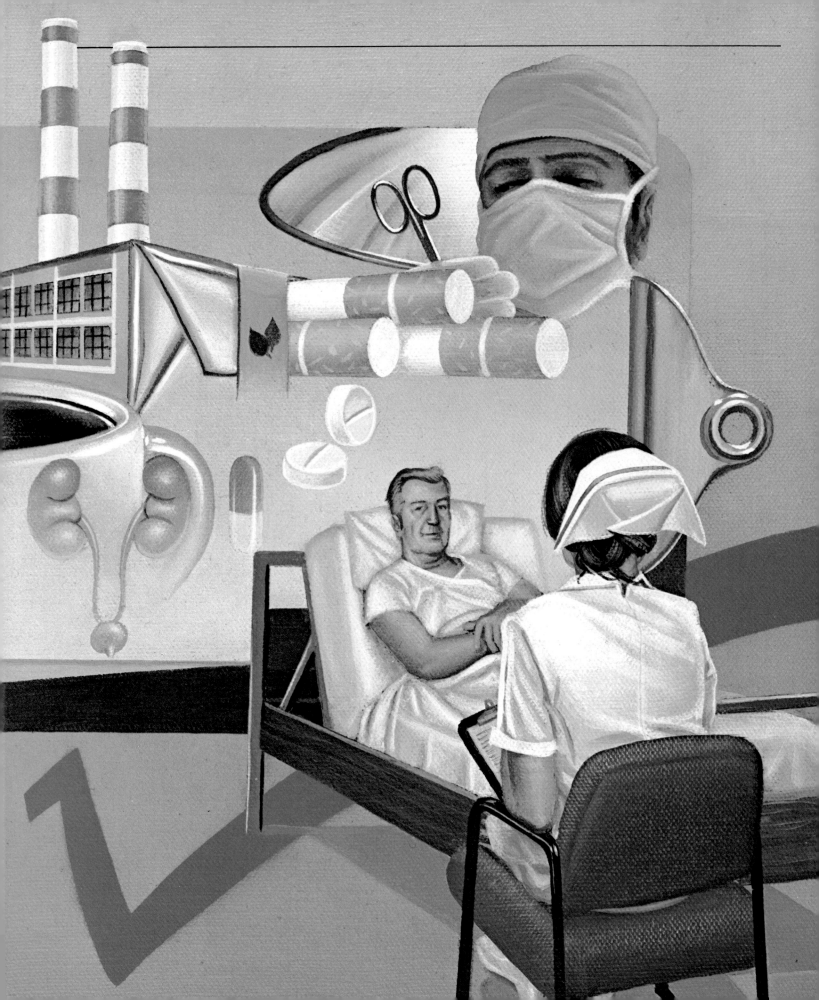

Patient assessment

Investigating urinary tract problems

When you question your patient about possible urologic problems, include questions about his reproductive system, because they may elicit significant information. Use this list as a guide. You may want to introduce and explore topics of your own.

Whether your patient's male or female, consider these questions:
- How many times a day do you urinate? Have you noticed an increase or decrease in your frequency of urination? Have you noticed an increase or decrease in the amount of your urine?
- When you urinate, do you ever have trouble starting the flow?
- Has your urine stream changed in size? If so, can you describe it?
- When you're finished urinating, does your bladder feel completely empty?
- Do you wake up at night needing to urinate? How often does this occur? Does it happen only when you drink an unusual amount of fluid before going to bed?
- Do you have any problems with your kidneys or bladder? If so, what kind? Have you had any kidney or bladder problems in the past; for example, an infection?
- Have you ever had kidney or bladder stones? If so, when? How were they treated?
- Do you ever have a burning sensation when you urinate? If so, how frequently?
- What color is your urine? Does it ever look red, brown, black, or dark amber?
- Have you ever had a kidney injury? If so, when? How was it treated?
- Have you ever had surgery on your bladder or kidneys? What kind of surgery did you have? How long ago was it?
- Do you ever have sores or ulcers on your genitals? If so, how often? Are they painful? Do they ooze or drain?
- Have you ever had syphilis, gonorrhea, or any other venereal disease? How long ago? How was it treated?
- Is your sexual life satisfying? Do you ever experience pain or discomfort during intercourse?

If your patient's a male, consider these additional questions:
- Are you circumcised or uncircumcised?
- If you're uncircumcised, do you have trouble retracting your foreskin? After it's retracted, can you easily return it to its normal position?
- Have you noticed a change in your penis' color? If so, describe it. Do you have any discharge from your penis? If so, when did you first notice it? What color is it?
- Are you able to obtain and sustain an erection? Have you noticed a change in your sex drive?
- Have you ever had problems with your testicles, such as pain or swelling?
- Have you ever been treated for a prostate problem?
- Have you ever had prostate surgery?
- Do you take medication to correct a hormonal imbalance?
- Can you describe any other problems?

If your patient's a female, consider these additional questions:
- Do you have a problem with urine leaking? If so, does it leak only when you laugh or cough?
- Do you retain fluid during your menstrual periods? Do your hands or feet ever swell?
- Are you pregnant now? Have you ever been pregnant? If so, how many times? Have you had any problems with your pregnancies?
- Do you practice birth control? If so, what method do you use? How long have you been using this method? Is it satisfactory?
- If you use birth-control pills, how long have you been taking them? What type of pill are you taking? Have you ever had any problems that may be associated with taking the pill; for example, a headache, localized pain in your calves or chest, or fluid retention? If so, describe them.
- Do you have any vaginal discharge? If so, describe it. Does any pain or itching accompany it?
- When did you have your last Pap smear? What were the results? Have the results of your Pap smear ever been abnormal?
- Have you ever had surgery on your uterus, fallopian tubes, or ovaries? Why was it necessary? How long has it been since your surgery?
- Do you have any other problems?

Assessing your patient's bladder and kidneys

1 *When you assess your patient's bladder and kidneys, you follow the same procedure regardless of your patient's sex.*

Begin by asking your patient to urinate, to ensure an empty bladder. Explain the assessment procedure and ask her to lie flat. Then, follow these steps:

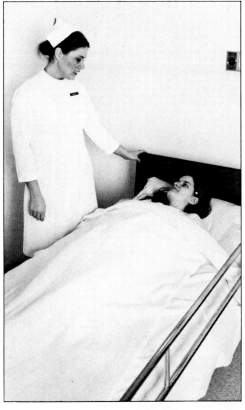

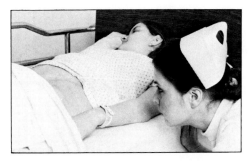

3 Suppose the retained urine is so great that the bladder's distended. You'll usually be able to see, at eye level, a swelling above the symphysis pubis.

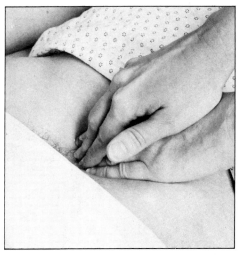

4 If the bladder's not distended, you may have difficulty locating it. Continue by deeply palpating the patient's abdomen, midline, about 1″ above her symphysis pubis. If you feel the rounded edge of the bladder, continue to palpate until you can estimate the bladder's location and size. Note any lumps, masses, or tenderness.

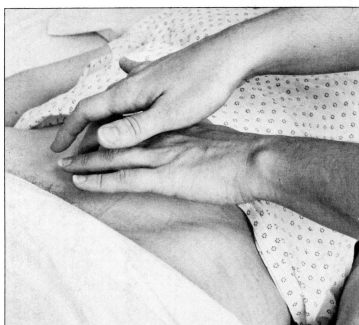

2 Percuss the area over her bladder, beginning about 2″ above the symphysis pubis and moving downward. You'll hear a tympanic sound if everything's okay. But if you hear a dull sound, the bladder has retained urine. Confirm this observation by palpating just above the symphysis pubis. If urine has been retained, the bladder will feel smooth and firm.

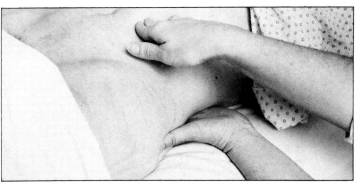

5 Now, here's how to assess your patient's kidneys. Place one hand underneath your patient, midway between her lower costal margin and iliac crest. Position your other hand on your patient's abdomen, also between the lower costal margin and iliac crest.

Now, press your hands together each time your patient inhales. Increase your pressure with each inhalation until you reach the maximum palpation depth.

At this point, tell your patient to inhale deeply. As she does, you should feel the lower pole of her kidney move down between your hands. Note the kidney's contour and size. It should be about 4¼″ long, 2″ to 3″ wide, and 1″ thick (10.8 cm long, 5 to 7.6 cm wide, and 2.5 cm thick). Also check for any lumps, masses, or tenderness.

Move your hands to your patient's other side. Palpate her other kidney in the same manner. Is one kidney significantly smaller than the other? If so, document your finding. Such a condition may indicate kidney malfunction.

Patient assessment

Assessing your patient's bladder and kidneys continued

6 Suppose you can't feel your patient's kidneys. Try using another palpation technique, known as capturing the kidney.

To do this, position your hands as before and instruct your patient to inhale deeply. At the peak of inhalation, quickly—but gently—press your hands together. Now, tell your patient to exhale as slowly as possible. After she's exhaled completely, slowly release your hands. As you do, you should feel your patient's kidney slide between your hands. Assess its size, contour, and any abnormalities.

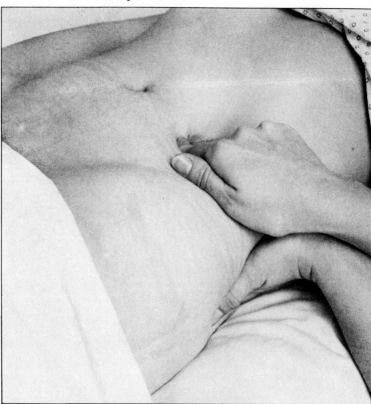

7 What if you can't feel your patient's kidneys using either of these palpation techniques? Then, try this method. Although it's not a regular assessment technique, you can use it to check for tenderness. Here's how:

Ask your patient to sit up. Place your palm on her back slightly to the right of her costovertebral angle, as shown in the large photo. Hit the back of your positioned hand with your fist, as shown in the inset. If your patient feels pain, she may have a kidney infection.

Repeat the procedure on your patient's other side.

Whatever method you use, document all findings in your nurses' notes.

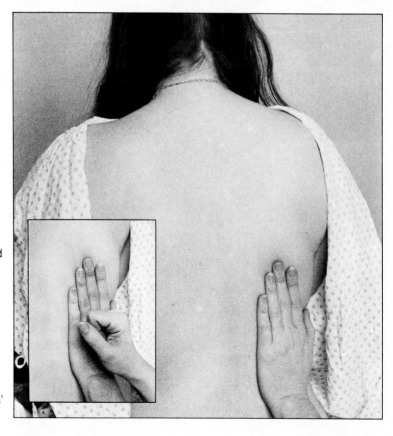

PATIENT TEACHING

Taking a urine specimen

You'll routinely request a urine specimen from all new urology patients. The collection procedure's not difficult, but the trick is to avoid contaminating the specimen.

In most cases, you'll instruct the patient how to obtain the specimen himself. As a guide, use the self-care aids on the pages that follow, and give your patient a copy. You might want to read it over with him, emphasizing the steps that minimize the chance of contamination. You'll also need to give him some disposable wipes and a specimen cup with a lid.

Your hospital may have bathroom dispensers of disposable wipes (presaturated with iodophor). If this is the case, give the patient the specimen cup and lid. Tell him where the tissue dispenser is located, and how he should moisten the tissues with water before use.

◢ *Nursing tip:* Post the self-care aids in the bathrooms where they can be read easily. This may increase the number of patients who follow your instructions.

If you suspect your patient has kidney stones, give him an unsterile graduated container in addition to the sterile specimen cup. Tell him he should not urinate into the toilet. Whatever urine he doesn't collect in the specimen cup, he should collect in the graduated container. Then, you can send the sterile specimen to the lab and pour the contents of the graduated container through a urine strainer funnel. If you detect any stones or stone particles, save them for the doctor to see. He may wish to send them to the lab for analysis.

Patient teaching

Self-care

Collecting a urine specimen (for the male patient)

1 Dear Patient:
Carefully follow these instructions for collecting a urine specimen. Doing so will help you avoid contaminating the specimen, which would interfere with the test results and necessitate repeating the procedure. Open the disposable wipe and place it on a nearby surface.

3 Remove the lid from the specimen cup and place it flat side down. Make sure you don't touch the inside of the lid.

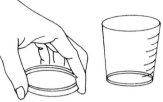

2 Prepare to urinate as you usually would. However, if you're uncircumcised, first pull back your foreskin. Using the disposable wipe, clean the head of your penis. Clean from the urethral opening toward you, as shown. Then, discard the wipe.

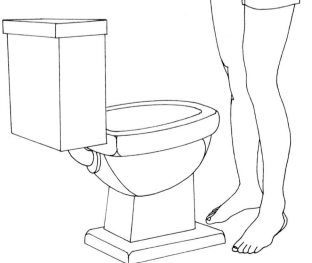

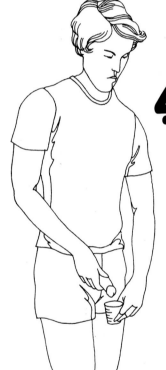

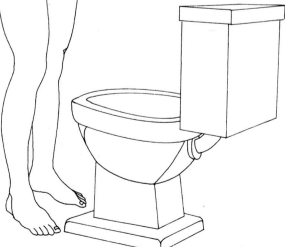

4 Urinate a small amount into the toilet or urinal; then, stop the flow. Hold the specimen cup a few inches away from your penis and finish urinating into the cup. But, don't let it overflow. Place the lid on the cup, and return the filled cup to the nurse.

Patient teaching

Self-care

Collecting a urine specimen (for the female patient)

1 Dear Patient:
Carefully follow these instructions for collecting a urine specimen. By doing so, you avoid contaminating the specimen, which would interfere with the test results and necessitate repeating the procedure. First, remove all your clothes from the waist down. Open the three disposable wipes and place them on a nearby surface.

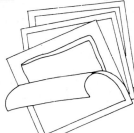

2 Sit as far back on the toilet as possible and spread apart your legs.

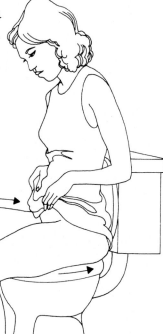

3 Remove the lid from the specimen cup and place it flat side down. Make sure you don't touch the inside of the lid.

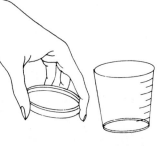

4 Using the fingers of one hand, separate your labia. Keep them separated for the rest of the procedure.

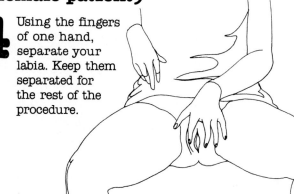

5 With the other hand, take one of the wipes and clean one side of the labia, using one stroke going from top to bottom. Discard the wipe. Take another and clean the other side of the labia. Again use only one stroke and discard the wipe afterwards. Then, take the last disposable wipe and clean the meatus. Discard this wipe also.

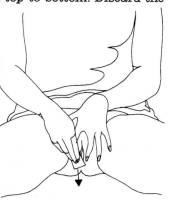

6 Urinate a small amount into the toilet. Then, hold the specimen cup a few inches from your urethra and finish urinating into the cup. But, don't let it overflow. Place the lid on the cup. Get dressed, and return the filled cup to the nurse.

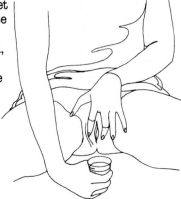

Patient assessment

Analyzing a urine specimen

After your patient's urine specimen goes to the lab for analysis, do you know what happens to it? The lab technician will usually test it for characteristics and levels detailed in this chart, in addition to any special tests the doctor may order.

Characteristic	Normal finding	Abnormal findings	Possible causes
Color	Pale yellow to dark amber (varies with concentration)	• Colorless	• Excessive fluid intake • Chronic renal disease • Diabetes insipidus
		• Cloudy white	• Parasitic disease
		• Yellow to amber with pinkish sediment	• Hyperuricemia and gout
		• Yellow to amber with whitish sediment	• Infection
		• Deep orange to orange-red	• Obstructive jaundice (false reasons include cascara sagrada, rhubarb, beets, senna)
		• Orange-red to red	• Hemoglobinuria • Malaria • Internal bleeding • Porphyria (false reasons include Pyridium, phenolphthalein, phenolsulfonphthalein [PSP] dye)
		• Green-blue to black	• Melanoma (false reasons include methylene blue medication)
Turbidity (lucidity)	Clear	• Cloudy	• Infection • Urinary tract disease (false reasons include presence of amorphous phosphate)
Specific gravity (concentration as compared with H_2O)	1.005 to 1.025 (varies with hydration level)	• Dilute (1.001 to 1.010) or concentrated (1.025 to 1.030) urine	• Low specific gravity may be caused by kidney disorders or diabetes insipidus. (False reasons for high specific gravity include presence of pus, albumin, contrast media, or dextran.)
Acidity (pH)	pH 4.8 to 7.5	• Greater than pH 7.5	• Renal acidosis • Calculi
Protein	Little to no protein	• Proteinuria	• Serious kidney or proximal tubule disorder • Toxemia • Severe heart failure
Glucose	None	• Glycosuria	• Gestational diabetes • Diabetes mellitus (false reasons include dextrose therapy)
Red blood cells	None to three/high-power field	• More than three/high-power field	• Kidney malfunction or trauma to the urinary tract • Tumor or infection in the urinary tract
White blood cells	None to four/high-power field	• More than four/high-power field	• Bacterial infection

Patient assessment

Taking a 24-hour urine specimen

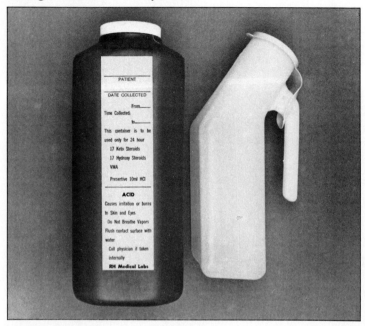

Many of the tests done for urinalysis involve chemical or hormonal quantities so small that they're microscopic. To deal with more measurable quantities, your patient's doctor may order a 24-hour urine collection. Here's how it's done:

On the morning the collection is to begin, instruct the patient to urinate into a graduated specimen container upon awakening. Record the time he does this; then measure the amount, and record it on the intake/output record. Discard the specimen.

Begin your 24-hour collection with the patient's second urine specimen. Ask him to urinate into a container. Record the time; then, measure and record the amount. Empty this container's contents into a 2500 ml bottle that's been properly labeled. Depending on what the doctor wants to study, the bottle may or may not contain a preservative, such as thymol crystals or toluene.

Important: If the bottle does contain a preservative, be careful not to splash any on your skin. To protect the patient from possible skin irritation, tell him not to urinate directly into the bottle.

Check with the laboratory to see if you should refrigerate the urine specimen. Also, find out if the doctor wants any diet or medication schedule changes made for the duration of the collection.

The final specimen of your 24-hour collection should be the patient's first specimen the following morning. If possible, collect it at the same time you began the collection procedure 24 hours earlier. Finally, record the time and amount of this specimen.

Analyzing a 24-hour urine specimen

On a 24-hour urine specimen, the lab will probably do several tests in addition to the ones done on a single urine specimen. This chart describes the most common of these tests. When you study it, note the creatinine clearance value. As you can see, this value isn't calculated over a 24- hour period, as the other values are. Instead, using the patient's body surface and age, it's an estimate of the amount of creatinine that the kidney can filter in 1 minute.

Test	Normal value	Implication of abnormality
Aldosterone	*Male and female:* 2 to 16 µg/24 hours	Increase indicates either nephrotic syndrome or adrenal malfunction.
17-hydroxycorticosteroids	*Male and female:* 3.8 mg/24 hours	Decrease indicates adrenocortical malfunction.
17-ketosteroids	*Male:* 6 to 21 mg/24 hours *Female:* 4 to 17 mg/24 hours	Increase indicates adrenal hyperplasia.
Catecholamines (norepinephrine, epinephrine, dopamine)	*Male and female:* Norepinephrine: 15 to 80 µg/24 hours Epinephrine: 0 to 20 µg/24 hours Dopamine: 65 to 400 µg/24 hours	Increase in any may indicate pheochromocytoma.
Calcium, phosphorous, and creatinine clearance	Calcium *Male:* less than 275 mg/24 hours *Female:* less than 250 mg/24 hours Phosphorus *Male and female:* less than 1,100 mg/24 hours Creatinine *Male:* 90 ml/min/1.73m² at age 20 *Female:* 84 ml/min/1.73m² at age 20 (Decrease by 6 ml/min/decade)	Increase in any indicates hyperparathyroidism, which can cause calculi.

Urologic blood tests: What they indicate

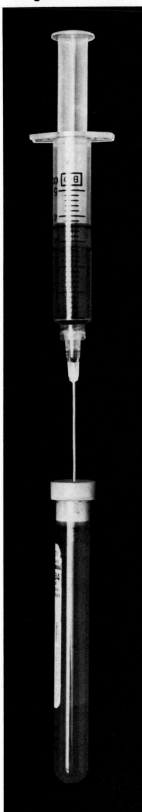

The doctor may order any number of blood tests for a newly admitted urology patient. The most important blood tests are listed below. The first six are part of a comprehensive study known as an SMA12. Other tests in this study are used to check for metastasized tissue and to determine serum electrolyte levels. The doctor will also order a complete blood count (CBC). A high white blood cell level indicates that your patient has an infection.

Test	Normal value	Implication of abnormality
Acid phosphatase	*Male and female:* 3 to 7 units/liter	High level may indicate metastatic carcinoma of the breast, hyperparathyroidism, renal insufficiency, and in the male patient, metastatic cancer of the prostate gland. (False high level occurs immediately after a rectal exam because of prostatic stimulation.)
Albumin	*Male and female:* 3.05 to 4.3 gram/100 ml	Low level may indicate renal failure.
Blood urea nitrogen (BUN)	*Male:* 17 to 51 mg/100 ml *Female:* 13 to 45 mg/100 ml	Increase may indicate renal impairment or obstruction, or shock or heart failure.
Calcium	*Male and female:* 8.9 to 10.1 mg/100 ml	Decrease may indicate the onset of renal failure.
Chloride	*Male and female:* 100 to 108 mEq/liter	Decrease may indicate the onset of renal failure.
Creatinine	*Male:* 0.8 to 1.2 mg/100 ml *Female:* 0.6 to 0.9 mg/100 ml	Increase may indicate renal damage or insufficiency.
Potassium	*Male and female:* 3.6 to 4.8 mEq/liter	Level is affected by dehydration that can be caused by renal treatments or renal impairment. If allowed to become excessive, cardiac arrhythmias may result.
Sodium	*Male and female:* 135 to 145 mEq/liter	Increase may indicate decreased renal function.
Total protein	*Male and female:* 6.6 to 7.9 gram/100 ml	Low level may indicate renal failure.
Uric acid	*Male:* 4.3 to 8.0 mg/100 ml *Female:* 2.3 to 6.0 mg/100 ml	High level may indicate renal failure.

Patient assessment

Understanding diagnostic urology tests

The doctor can perform a multitude of diagnostic tests to help determine what's wrong with your patient's urinary tract. Exactly which tests he selects depends on a variety of information, including the patient's signs, symptoms, blood and urine test findings, and assessment findings.

You probably won't help perform these tests. But you should know what each involves so you can adequately prepare the patient for them. We've selected the ten most commonly performed tests to feature here. Since procedures may vary slightly from hospital to hospital, you should learn your hospital's specific requirements for each procedure.

Note: The doctor may decide against these tests if your patient's pregnant. All of the tests, except ultrasound, are invasive or involve exposure to radiation.

Type of test	Purpose	What to tell the patient
Computerized tomography (CT scan)	To evaluate the hard-to-visualize kidney; to identify structural abnormalities; to diagnose kidney or bladder mass.	You'll go to the X-ray room and lie down. The doctor or technician will position the arm of the X-ray machine over your body. Then, he'll send an X-ray beam through your body. The beam will be absorbed or deflected by your body's internal structures and then be recorded by a detector on the other side of your body. Next, the doctor or technician will move the scan arm slightly and repeat the procedure. Eventually the CT scan computer will have enough data to form a 3-dimensional view of your urologic structures. This will help the doctor diagnose your problem.
Cystography	To assess bladder function and explore the possible presence of stones in the bladder.	Your doctor may order a laxative the night before the test to clear out your intestinal system and make it easier to see. You won't be allowed to eat anything after that. In the morning you'll be taken to the X-ray room. The doctor will use a syringe to inject an anesthetic lubricant into your urethra to lubricate and numb it so you don't feel the tube. Then, he'll insert a flexible metal tube into your bladder and inject a dye through it. This dye can be seen when the doctor uses the X-ray machine. Several X-rays will be taken at 30 minute intervals. Then, the doctor will remove the tube and ask you to empty your bladder. If he takes X-rays while you do this, then he's also running a test called a voiding cystography. The X-rays from both tests will help the doctor determine how well your bladder works.
Cystometrography	To evaluate the motor and sensory functions of the bladder.	You'll go to the cystoscopy room. There you'll be positioned with your legs apart and knees bent so the doctor can insert a tube called a cystometer into your bladder. This monitor enables the doctor to measure your bladder pressure. To do this, he'll let sterile water or a sterile saltwater solution flow into your bladder. You'll be asked to tell the doctor when you feel you have to urinate. The doctor may continue to instill solution until your urge to urinate becomes involuntary. When that happens, he'll remove the tube so you can empty your bladder.
Intravenous pyelography	To assess kidney function and detect obstructions in the urinary tract. *Important:* Contraindicated for patient allergic to shellfish or iodine.	I'll give you a laxative the night before the test to clear out your intestinal system and make it easier for the doctor to see. You won't be allowed to eat or drink anything after that. Then, in the morning you'll be taken to the X-ray room. The doctor will use a syringe to inject a dye into a vein in your arm. For a few minutes after this dye enters your bloodstream, you'll experience hot flushing and a burning sensation. Before long, the dye will reach your kidneys. As it floods through them, the X-ray machine will take pictures of its path. Eventually, the dye will flow to your bladder for excretion. The entire test takes about 45 minutes.

Type of test	Purpose	What to tell the patient
Panendoscopy or cystoscopy	To judge the degree of bladder obstruction from an enlarged prostate or urethral stricture; to identify a polyp or tumor; to take a sterile urine sample; to take a prostate, bladder, or urethral biopsy; and to remove foreign bodies.	Before you're brought to the cystoscopy room of the surgical department, you may be given a sedative. Then, once you get there, you'll be placed on your back with your legs apart and knees bent. The doctor will inject anesthetic lubricant into your urethra to lubricate and numb it so you don't feel the tube. Then, he'll insert a panendoscope or cystoscope into your bladder to observe its internal structure. After he's done this, he'll record his findings and remove the instrument. Following the procedure, you may feel a burning sensation when you urinate, or have a little blood in your urine. Drinking water will help correct these side effects. *Note:* If the patient will remain in your unit, check his meatus for bleeding every hour for the first 24-hours after this procedure. If bleeding becomes excessive, notify the doctor.
Renography	To assess blood flow to the kidney and tubular function of the kidney.	You'll go to the X-ray room and sit in a chair that has no back. The doctor will place one renogram probe over each kidney and possibly a third below both kidneys. Then, he'll inject a dye into your arm and turn on the machine. For a few minutes following the injection, expect to feel a burning sensation. The machine will detect the dye passing in and out of your kidneys and produce a graph of the blood flow. This will help the doctor determine the condition of your kidneys.
Ultrasound	To diagnose the possibility of a peritoneal abscess, retroperitoneal mass, or a hemorrhage; to evaluate the success of a renal transplant; and to aid in a percutaneous kidney biopsy.	You'll be positioned lying down with your abdomen uncovered. The doctor or technician will place a disc called a transducer on your abdomen. The transducer will emit a narrow beam of sound waves into your body. The sound waves will hit your body's internal structures and bounce back to the transducer. The transducer's connected to a machine that will pick up the returning sound waves and convert them into an image on a TV-like screen called an oscilloscope. The doctor can use this image to help him diagnose abnormalities in your urinary tract.
Urethrography	To visualize abnormalities in the urethra.	You'll go to the X-ray room and lie down. The doctor will inject an anesthetic lubricant into your urethra to lubricate and numb it so you don't feel the tube. Then, he'll insert a flexible metal tube into your urethra and inject a dye into the tube. The radiologist will take several X-rays so your doctor can visualize the condition of your urethra.
Voiding cystourethrography	To visualize the ureters, bladder, and urethra, and demonstrate their function.	You'll be taken to the X-ray room. The doctor or technician will take several preliminary X-rays. Then, the doctor will use a syringe to inject a dye into your urethra. After waiting about 5 minutes, he'll take more X-rays. Then, he'll ask you to empty your bladder. Immediately after you do this, he'll take another X-ray. The X-rays will help him identify obstructions or help evaluate how well your urinary tract functions.

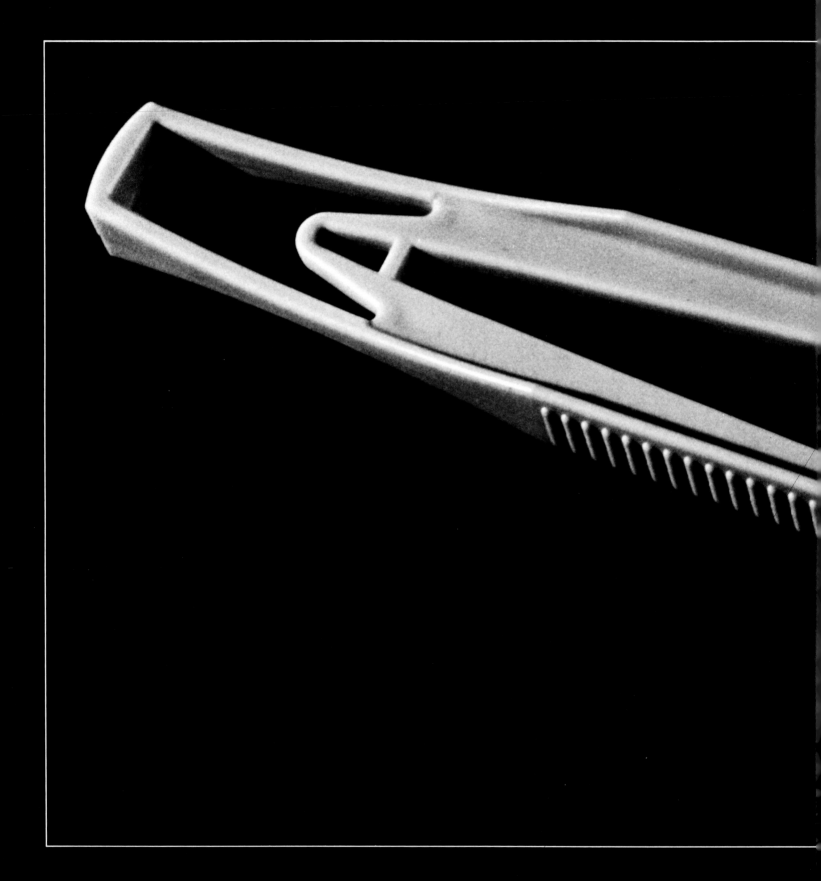

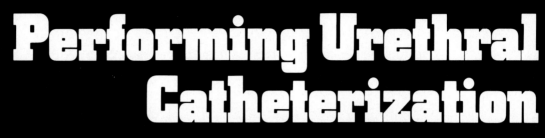

Performing Urethral Catheterization

Catheterization basics
Straight catheterization
Indwelling catheterization
Catheterization self-care

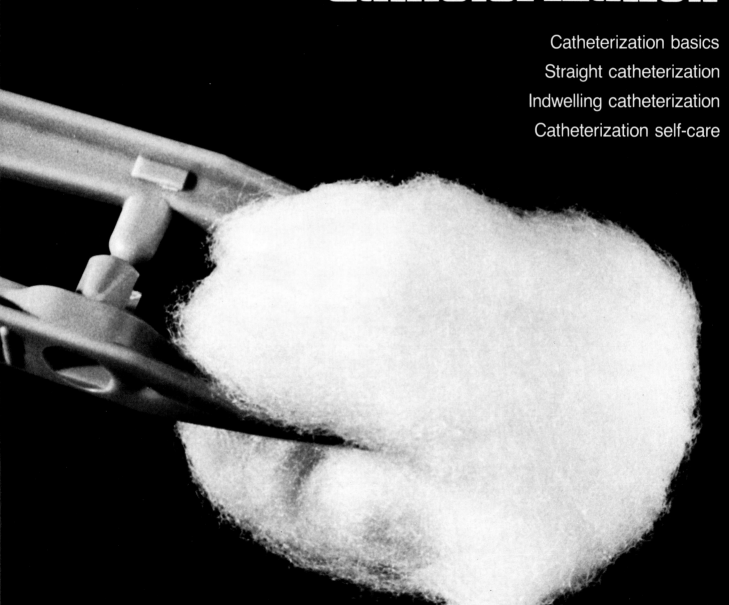

Catheterization basics

You probably know a number of reasons for performing catheterization. But we can also give you a few reasons why you shouldn't. Because catheterization can cause urethral trauma and introduce bacteria into the patient's urinary tract, avoid it whenever possible. For example, suppose you need a urine specimen. Don't catheterize your patient if you can teach him the clean-catch technique.

If you must catheterize your patient, your rule of thumb should be: the quicker, the better. The less time you let the catheter remain in your patient, the less chance you take of infecting him. So, one-time catheterization's better than intermittent catheterization and intermittent catheterization's better than indwelling catheterization. The reasons the doctor chooses one method of catheterization over another differ. To learn how they differ, read the chart to the right. Then, to discover how to perform each method, read the pages that follow.

Understanding different urethral catheterization methods

When you care for a patient with a urologic problem, do you wonder why the doctor has chosen straight catheterization or indwelling catheterization? To understand, you must know the indications for each method. Use this chart to decide why the doctor has chosen one method instead of another, as well as to determine what equipment is required. Note the nursing considerations column. It provides you with special information you should know for each method.

Method	Indications for use	Catheter description
Straight (one-time or intermittent)	*One-time:* • To relieve urine retention • To collect a sterile urine specimen • To determine presence of residual urine *Intermittent:* • To relieve urine retention • To collect a sterile urine specimen • To determine presence of residual urine • To control urinary incontinence	Robinson: a straight catheter with one or more openings near its tip. The tip comes in several styles, the most common ones being rounded and coudé.
Indwelling (continuous)	• To relieve urine retention • To monitor urine output • To provide postsurgical urine drainage • To permit bladder irrigation • To act as a stent (support) or hemostatic device after urologic surgery	Foley: a double- or triple-lumen catheter, with an inflatable balloon and a rounded tip. The double-lumen catheter also comes with a coudé tip.

Catheter variations	Nursing considerations
Robinson with rounded tip 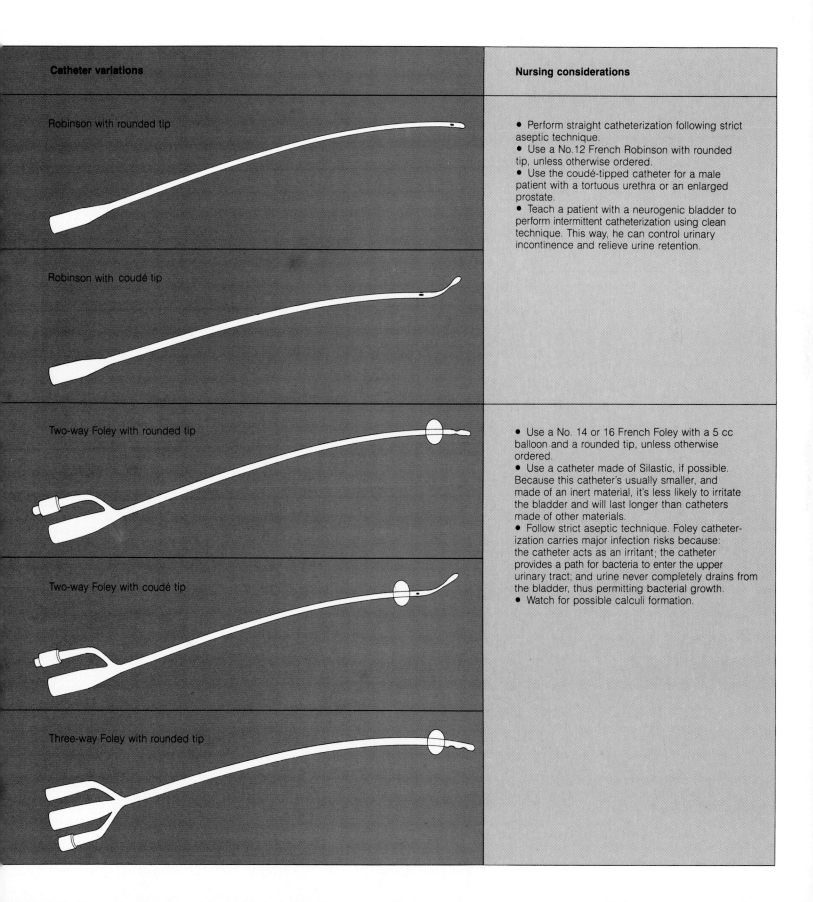	• Perform straight catheterization following strict aseptic technique. • Use a No. 12 French Robinson with rounded tip, unless otherwise ordered. • Use the coudé-tipped catheter for a male patient with a tortuous urethra or an enlarged prostate. • Teach a patient with a neurogenic bladder to perform intermittent catheterization using clean technique. This way, he can control urinary incontinence and relieve urine retention.
Robinson with coudé tip	
Two-way Foley with rounded tip	• Use a No. 14 or 16 French Foley with a 5 cc balloon and a rounded tip, unless otherwise ordered. • Use a catheter made of Silastic, if possible. Because this catheter's usually smaller, and made of an inert material, it's less likely to irritate the bladder and will last longer than catheters made of other materials. • Follow strict aseptic technique. Foley catheterization carries major infection risks because: the catheter acts as an irritant; the catheter provides a path for bacteria to enter the upper urinary tract; and urine never completely drains from the bladder, thus permitting bacterial growth. • Watch for possible calculi formation.
Two-way Foley with coudé tip	
Three-way Foley with rounded tip	

Straight catheterization

Straight catheterization's one of those basic procedures you perform almost every day. But just because catheterization's common, don't underestimate the importance of doing it correctly. For information about aseptic technique and the most comfortable insertion practices for your patient, read on.

In the next few pages, we'll tell you the correct way to insert a straight catheter in either a male or a female patient. These procedures include tips on:
- how to prepare your patient
- how to cope with common insertion problems
- how to position your patient, including a patient who's elderly or who can't lie on his back
- how to thoroughly prep the meatal area
- how to bypass obstructions and when not to try
- how to obtain a sterile urine specimen.

Inserting a straight catheter into a female patient

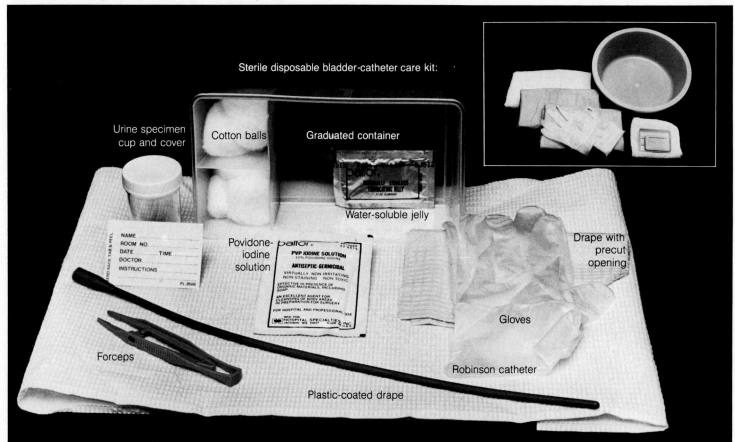

Sterile disposable bladder-catheter care kit:

Urine specimen cup and cover

Cotton balls

Graduated container

Water-soluble jelly

Povidone-iodine solution

Drape with precut opening

Gloves

Forceps

Robinson catheter

Plastic-coated drape

1 *Jane Smith, a 28-year-old teacher, is a postpartum patient who can't urinate after the birth of her child. So, the doctor orders intermittent catheterization every 6 to 8 hours. Do you know how to catheterize Mrs. Smith?*

To begin, review the patient's chart, paying particular attention to information concerning her urinary tract. For example, does your patient have a history of urinary tract infection? Also, carefully read the doctor's orders and determine the size of the catheter to be used. Usually, the doctor will order a No. 12 French Robinson catheter. (For comparison of catheter types, see pages 24 and 25.)

Now, make sure you gather everything pictured above, and place it at the patient's bedside.

The lubricating jelly shown here comes in a packet, but your kit

may provide jelly in a prefilled syringe. Some catheter care kits contain a No. 12 Robinson catheter, as well.

For washing your patient, obtain the equipment shown in the inset: clean examining gloves, two bed-saver pads, washcloth, basin, towel, soap, and warm water.

Make sure you have strong, direct lighting before you begin the procedure. A gooseneck lamp will help, if one's available.

Reassure your patient and explain what you're going to do. Remember, since catheterization involves the genitals, your patient may feel embarrassed. Protect her privacy by drawing the curtain around the bed or closing the door.

Remember to wash your hands before and after the procedure.

2 If possible, position your patient flat on her back, with her knees bent and her legs abducted, as shown here. Put a bed-saver pad under her buttocks. Place her feet 24″ (61 cm) apart.

If your patient is elderly—or for any reason, can't lie on her back—catheterize her lying on her side with her upper leg drawn up, knee to chest (Sims' position). With her legs in this position, you'll have good access to her perineum. Direct the light toward the perineal area.

3 Now, put on the clean examining gloves. Using a washcloth, wash the perineum with warm water and mild soap. Pat the area dry with a towel. Then, replace the wet bed-saver pad with a dry one. Remove your gloves.

Place the sterile catheter kit between your patient's legs (or behind them if she's in Sims' position). Open the kit, using aseptic technique. Then, if the Robinson catheter's packaged separately, open the package and drop the catheter into the open kit.

4 Now, put on the sterile gloves. Pull on the first glove by tucking the fingers of one hand into the glove's turned-up cuff, as shown here. Then, place the fingers of your gloved hand in the cuff of the second glove and pull on the second glove, as shown in the inset. At this point, loosen the specimen cup cap. Open the packets of cleansing solution and lubricating jelly.

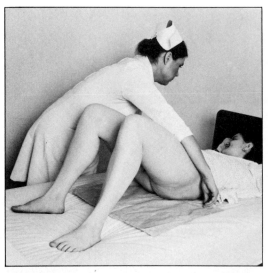

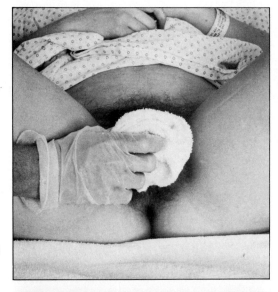

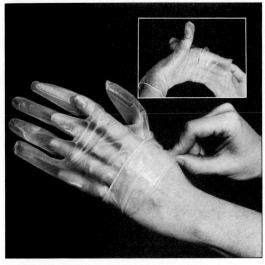

5 So you don't contaminate your gloved hands, pick up the plastic-coated drape and fold it over your hands, as shown here.

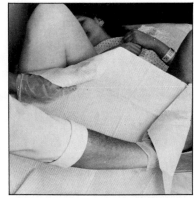

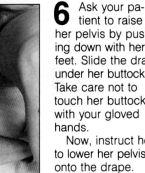

6 Ask your patient to raise her pelvis by pushing down with her feet. Slide the drape under her buttocks. Take care not to touch her buttocks with your gloved hands.

Now, instruct her to lower her pelvis onto the drape.

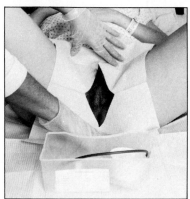

7 Next, position the precut drape so that the opening's over your patient's perineal area.

8 Pour solution over all the cotton balls except one. Later, you'll use the dry cotton ball to blot excess antiseptic from the meatus.

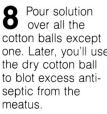

Straight catheterization

Inserting a straight catheter into a female patient continued

9 Next, squeeze the lubricating jelly onto the tray. Then, lubricate the first 3" (7.6 cm) of the catheter by rolling it in the jelly.

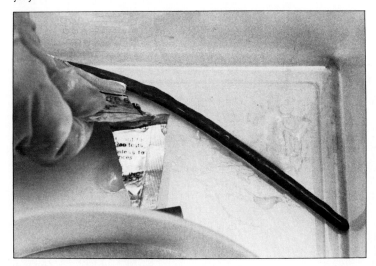

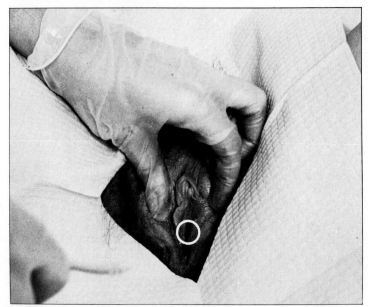

10 Now, you're ready to clean your patient's perineal area. First, use your nondominant hand to spread apart the patient's labia. Separate the labia with your thumb and index finger. This will help expose the patient's urethral meatus.

Be extremely careful not to confuse the patient's urethral opening with her vaginal opening. Look for the meatus between her clitoris and vagina. If you can't see it, it may be hidden in the anterior part of the vagina. If you can't find it there, try exerting a slight downward pressure when you clean between the labia (see step 11). This should open the meatus briefly.

For an obese patient, ask an assistant to hold the labial folds during the entire catheterization procedure, so you can see the meatus.

Important: The hand used to spread apart the labia is now contaminated. Don't use it to insert the catheter.

11 With your uncontaminated hand, use the forceps to pick up a saturated cotton ball. By doing this, you keep the hand sterile for catheter insertion. With a downward stroke, clean the right labia minora, as shown.

To preserve the sterile field, discard the cotton ball into a waste basket. Use another saturated cotton ball to clean the left labia minora. Discard this cotton ball, too. Repeat the procedure, once more, stroking down the middle between the labia minora.

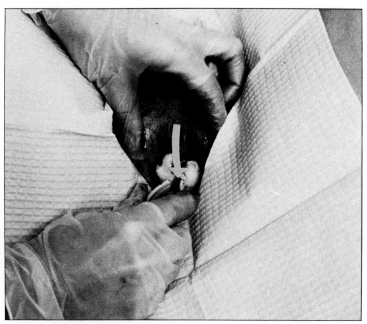

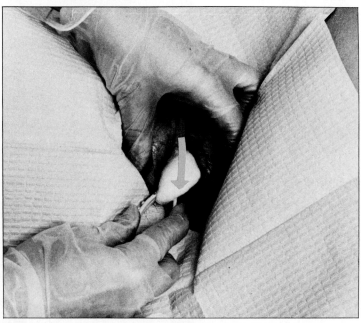

12 Now, holding one of the dry cotton balls in the forceps, make one last stroke between the labia. This will blot any excess antiseptic. Be sure no wisps of cotton remain on the perineum.

13 Now, you're ready to begin insertion. Grasp the Robinson catheter with your uncontaminated hand, as you would a pencil or a dart. This will give you greater control. Making sure you don't touch the catheter to the unprepped areas of the perineum, gently insert it 2″ to 3″ (5 to 7.6 cm) into the meatus. Angle the catheter slightly upward as you advance it. Note: Never force the catheter.

If your patient displays discomfort, encourage her to relax, exhale, and inhale deeply. While she's inhaling, advance the catheter. A deep inhalation relaxes the external sphincter muscle and can ease the catheter's passage. If it still won't pass easily, try a smaller catheter. If a smaller catheter won't pass, call the doctor. *Important:* If you must break aseptic technique to introduce a smaller catheter, obtain a new kit and start again.

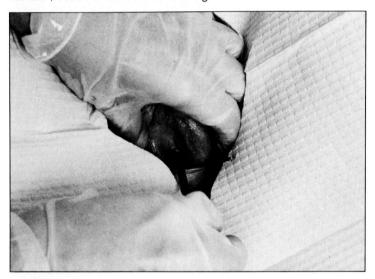

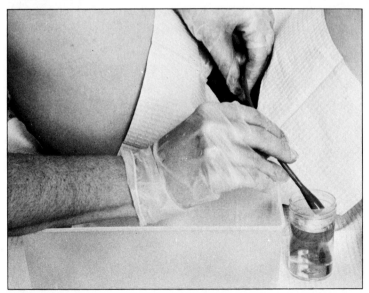

14 As the catheter enters the patient's bladder, urine will begin draining. Release the labia. Using your sterile hand, place the free end of the catheter in the specimen container. Make sure you grasp the catheter high enough to avoid contaminating the specimen. Let the container fill to the three-quarters mark.

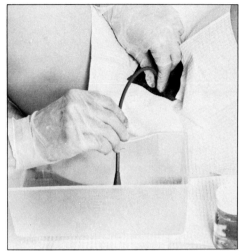

15 Empty the bladder by draining the remaining urine into the kit's graduated container. But, be careful. Don't allow more than 700 ml urine to drain into the container. If the urine reaches this level, clamp the catheter immediately. Allowing more than 700 ml urine to drain at one time may cause your patient to go into shock.

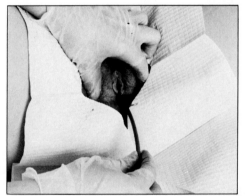

16 When you're finished, gently pinch the catheter and remove it. Pinching the catheter prevents urine from leaking into the urethra. Discard the catheter.

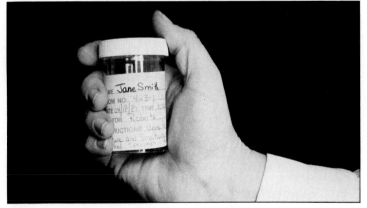

17 Examine the urine specimen. In your nurses' notes, document the amount of urine, its color, and its lucidity. Note any sediment, odor, or blood clots. Start an intake/output record, remembering to include the amount of urine in the specimen. Label the specimen with the patient's name, her room number, her hospital identification number, the doctor's name, and the date. Indicate that you obtained the specimen by catheter. Attach a lab slip and send the specimen to the lab immediately. Remember, the fresher the specimen, the more accurate the lab results will be.

Record on the patient's care plan how she tolerated catheterization.

Straight catheterization

Inserting a straight catheter in a male patient

1 *You may work in a hospital that prohibits catheterization of male patients by female nurses. But, suppose your hospital changes its policy. If a doctor instructs you to catheterize a male patient to relieve postoperative urinary retention, will you know what to do?*

As you read this story about catheterization of males, refer to the preceding story on catheterization of females for more details.

First, review the patient's chart and the doctor's orders. Be sure to ask the patient whether he's been catheterized previously. If so, was the catheterization difficult? If the patient says yes, consult a doctor. The patient may have *deep bulb false passages,* which are channels formed by a sharp-tipped urinary catheter during forceful insertion. Or the patient may have urethral strictures. You

may need to obtain a coudé catheter to help bypass these obstructions.

Assemble the same equipment that you gathered for female catheterization, as shown below. Some catheter care kits contain a No. 12 French Robinson catheter. The lubricating jelly may come in a packet, or in a syringe, for direct injection into the male patient's urethra.

For washing the patient, obtain this additional equipment: clean examining gloves, two bed-saver pads, washcloth, basin, towel, soap, and warm water.

Explain the procedure to your patient and take steps to protect his privacy. Then, wash your hands.

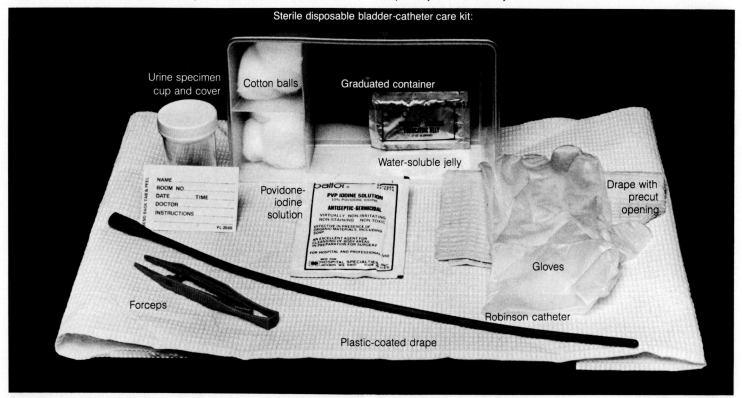

Sterile disposable bladder-catheter care kit:

Urine specimen cup and cover

Cotton balls

Graduated container

Water-soluble jelly

NAME
ROOM NO.
DATE   TIME
DOCTOR
INSTRUCTIONS

Povidone-iodine solution

PVP IODINE SOLUTION

Drape with precut opening

Gloves

Forceps

Robinson catheter

Plastic-coated drape

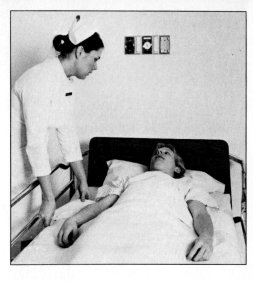

2 Position the patient flat on his back, if possible. Place the bed-saver pad under his buttocks.

If your patient can't lie on his back, have him lie on his side, sit on the edge of the bed, or stand.

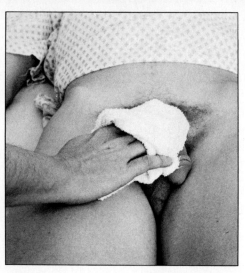

3 Wash the patient's penis and perineal area with soap and water; then pat dry. Replace the wet bed-saver pad with a new one.

4 Open the catheter care kit, the catheter package, and the packets of antiseptic solution and lubricating jelly, using aseptic technique. But don't put the equipment between the patient's legs. With a male patient, you'll work from a bedside table or overbed stand.

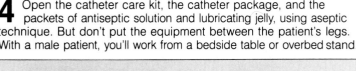

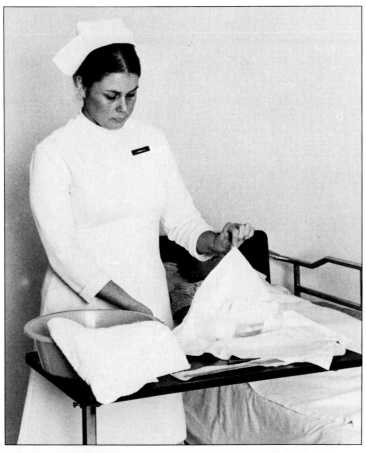

6 Now, pick up the precut drape with your normal working hand. With the other hand, guide the patient's penis through the opening in the drape. Consider this hand contaminated. Position the drape as shown.

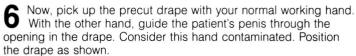

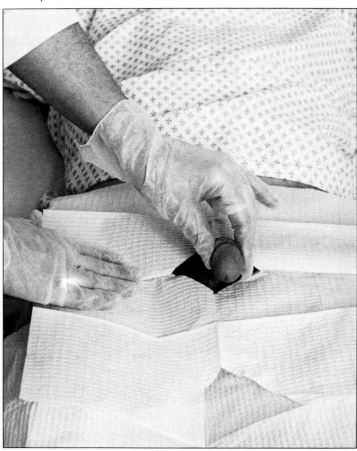

5 Put on sterile gloves, using the technique described on page 27. Now you're ready to drape your patient. Fold the plastic-coated drape over your gloved hands, as shown here, so that you don't contaminate your hands. Place the drape across your patient's thighs, as shown in the inset.

7 Now you're ready to clean the meatal area. Using your uncontaminated hand, pour antiseptic over all but one cotton ball. You'll save this cotton ball for drying.

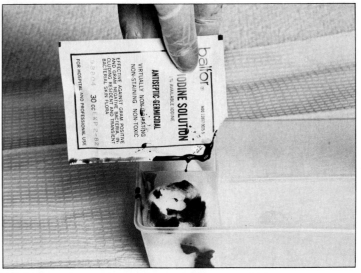

Straight catheterization

Inserting a straight catheter in a male patient continued

8 Then, take the patient's penis in your contaminated hand. [Inset] If your patient's uncircumcised, pull back his foreskin with the same hand.

With your uncontaminated hand, use the forceps to pick up a povidone-iodine saturated cotton ball. Clean around the meatus, using a circular motion. Then, clean in a spiral motion to the corona of the glans penis. Repeat this cleaning process with each saturated cotton ball. When all of them are used, discard them into the wastebasket, not on the sterile field. Blot any excess antiseptic from the penis with the dry cotton ball. Check to make sure no wisps of cotton remain on the penis.

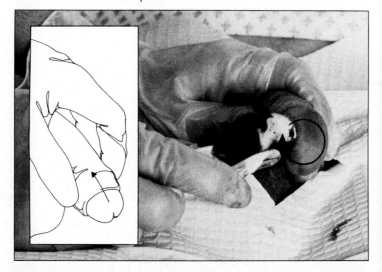

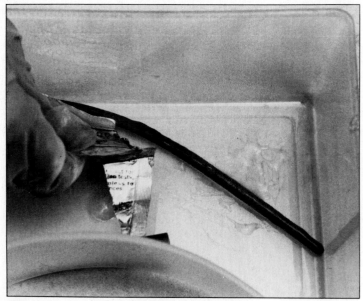

9 Using your uncontaminated hand, generously lubricate the first 7″ to 10″ (17.8 to 25.4 cm) of the catheter. Ample lubrication's particularly important for a male patient. If your kit contains a prefilled syringe of lubricating jelly, rather than a packet, inject all 10 ml jelly into the meatus. Then, remove the syringe and gently squeeze the area around the meatus to prevent the lubricant from oozing out.

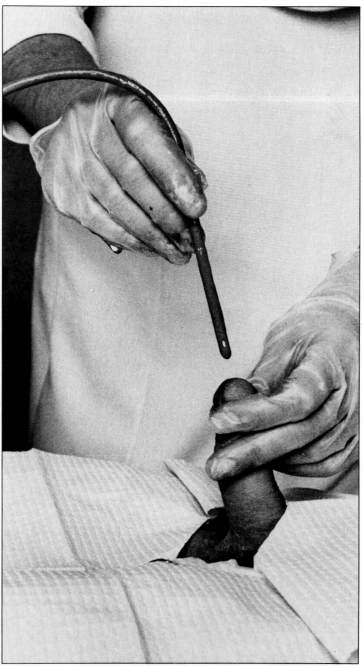

10 To prepare for insertion, hold the penis at a 90° angle to the patient's thighs. Grasp the catheter with your uncontaminated hand, as though it were a pencil or a dart, and gently insert the catheter into the meatus. Lower the penis to a 60° angle. This position changes the curve of the urethra from an S shape to a more relaxed curve, making catheter passage easier.

Advance the catheter 7″ to 10″ (17.8 cm to 25.4 cm) along the anterior wall of the urethra. A few inches into the urethra (at the external sphincter, which is just below the prostate), you'll encounter resistance from most patients. If your patient shows discomfort, reassure him. Ask him to exhale, then to inhale deeply. Advance the catheter during his deep inhalation.

11 Suppose, during insertion, that the catheter springs back an inch or two when you momentarily release it, or that it bends inside the penis. Assume you've encountered an obstruction. If this happens at the external sphincter, try increasing traction on the penis while gently advancing the catheter.

If you encounter an obstruction about 6″ (15.2 cm) into an elderly male's urethra, suspect prostate gland enlargement. In this case, try twisting and advancing the catheter, with the penis fully extended, or reduce the angle of the penis. Deep breathing will help the patient endure any discomfort he feels while you're trying to bypass an obstruction.

Important: Never forcibly insert a catheter. If you can't bypass an obstruction by gentle maneuvering, call the doctor. The doctor will introduce the catheter, using a guide. If that proves unsuccessful, he'll probably dilate the urethra after putting the patient under general anesthesia.

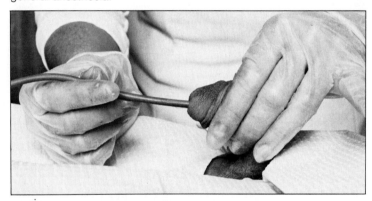

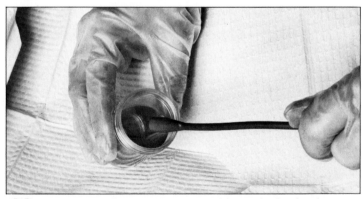

12 When the catheter enters the bladder and urine begins to flow, take a specimen as you would from a catheterized female. Always take a urine specimen when you catheterize a patient, unless you've taken one within the past 6 hours.

Then, empty the bladder by draining the remaining urine into your kit's graduated container. But never drain more than 700 ml at one time, or your patient may go into shock.

When you're finished, pinch the catheter and remove it slowly. Pinching the catheter will prevent urine from leaking into the urethra. Discard the catheter.

Note: After catheter removal, be sure to pull the foreskin forward on an uncircumcised male. If left retracted, the foreskin will impede circulation, causing painful swelling. Call the doctor immediately if you can't pull the foreskin back to its normal position.

Document the procedure as you would for female catheterization, and send the properly labeled specimen to the lab.

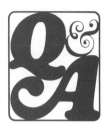

Coping with common insertion problems

Now you know how to insert a catheter. But insertion may not always go smoothly. Here are some answers to your questions about common problems.

What if the patient's combative or delirious?

Get assistance. Have three helpers gently restrain the patient—one holding his hands and two holding his legs.

What if the patient's obese?

A male patient's penis may be hidden in his fat folds. Make a vee with your index finger and thumb and apply pressure inward and upward around his penis. This should force out the penis so that you can prep and catheterize it.

With a female patient, have an assistant hold the labia apart during the catheterization procedure.

What if the patient has an erection?

Continue with the procedure. Reassure him that there's no harm in catheterizing his penis while it's erect. Usually a penis will become detumescent when you introduce a catheter into the meatus.

What if the catheter won't drain?

If the catheter won't drain at first insertion, the urine flow may be occluded by lubricant. Apply gentle suprapubic pressure to clear the lubricant and establish drainage.

If the catheter still won't drain, the patient's bladder may be empty. Wait several minutes. Still no drainage? Remove the catheter and irrigate it to check its patency. Doing this will determine if the problem's with the equipment or with the patient. In either case, obtain a new catheter and kit, and repeat the insertion procedure. If the second catheter won't drain, inform the doctor immediately.

What if I see blood during or after the catheterization procedure?

Stop the procedure and call the doctor immediately.

Indwelling catheterization

How often have you inserted an indwelling urethral catheter? Several times? Many times? If you've done it more than once, you may feel that you understand insertion well enough. But do you know the full range of procedures involved in catheter care after insertion? For example, do you know:
• how to aspirate a urine specimen?
• how to empty a leg bag?
• how to irrigate the catheter?
• how to connect a urine meter to the catheter?
• how to remove the catheter?

If you're familiar with indwelling catheterization, you probably realize the risk of infection involved with this method. But you may not fully understand the importance of strict aseptic technique in catheter insertion and care. Where catheter-induced infection's concerned, minor precautions can make a big difference. For example, you can help prevent infection by washing your hands before you touch any part of the catheter system, and by swabbing the drain tube with povidone-iodine solution when you empty the drainage bag. But these are just a few of the tips we'll give you in the following pages.

Read these pages to find out everything you need to know for aseptic catheter insertion and conscientious catheter care. Note that you always use a Foley catheter for indwelling urethral catheterization. Read the information about the Foley several times over. Practice the recommended measures, and you'll soon make them a natural part of your patient's care.

Using a closed drainage system to prevent infection

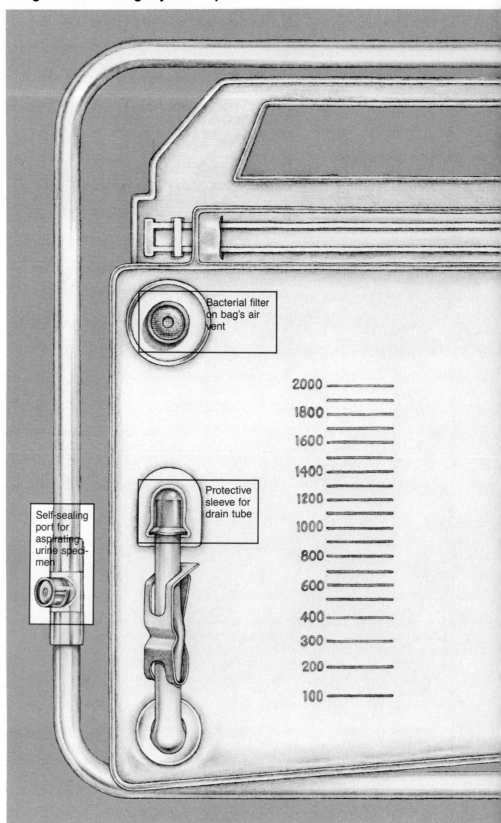

Bacterial filter on bag's air vent

Self-sealing port for aspirating urine specimen

Protective sleeve for drain tube

2000
1800
1600
1400
1200
1000
800
600
400
300
200
100

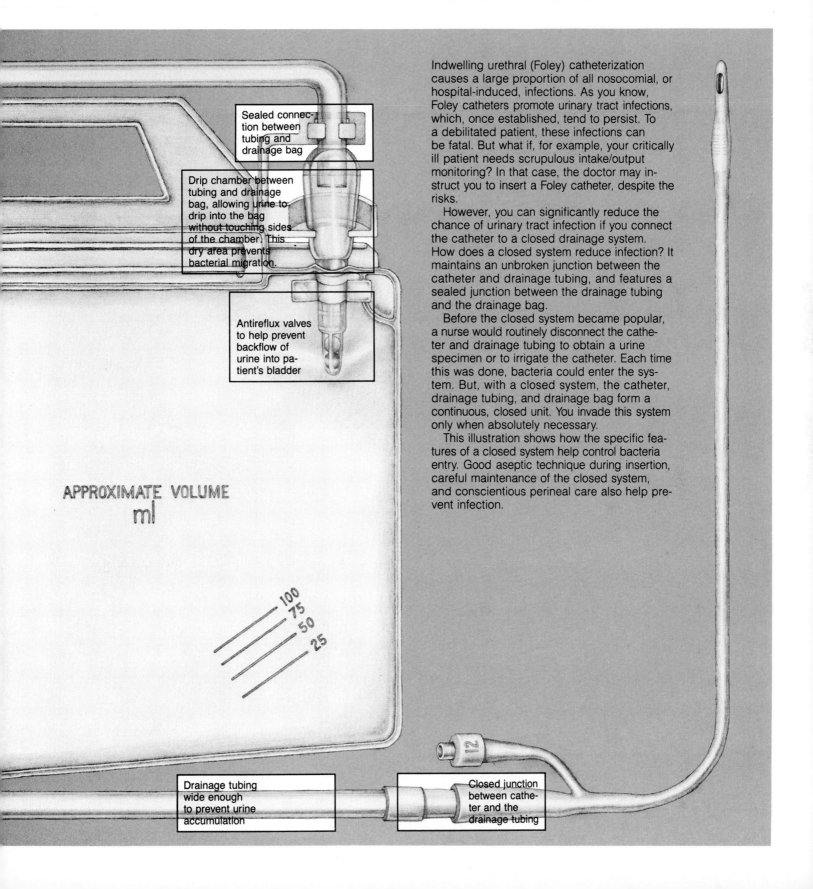

Sealed connection between tubing and drainage bag

Drip chamber between tubing and drainage bag, allowing urine to drip into the bag without touching sides of the chamber. This dry area prevents bacterial migration.

Antireflux valves to help prevent backflow of urine into patient's bladder

APPROXIMATE VOLUME
ml

100
75
50
25

Drainage tubing wide enough to prevent urine accumulation

Closed junction between catheter and the drainage tubing

Indwelling urethral (Foley) catheterization causes a large proportion of all nosocomial, or hospital-induced, infections. As you know, Foley catheters promote urinary tract infections, which, once established, tend to persist. To a debilitated patient, these infections can be fatal. But what if, for example, your critically ill patient needs scrupulous intake/output monitoring? In that case, the doctor may instruct you to insert a Foley catheter, despite the risks.

However, you can significantly reduce the chance of urinary tract infection if you connect the catheter to a closed drainage system. How does a closed system reduce infection? It maintains an unbroken junction between the catheter and drainage tubing, and features a sealed junction between the drainage tubing and the drainage bag.

Before the closed system became popular, a nurse would routinely disconnect the catheter and drainage tubing to obtain a urine specimen or to irrigate the catheter. Each time this was done, bacteria could enter the system. But, with a closed system, the catheter, drainage tubing, and drainage bag form a continuous, closed unit. You invade this system only when absolutely necessary.

This illustration shows how the specific features of a closed system help control bacteria entry. Good aseptic technique during insertion, careful maintenance of the closed system, and conscientious perineal care also help prevent infection.

Indwelling catheterization

Inserting a Foley catheter into a female patient

1 *Twenty-four hours after you began catheterizing her intermittently, Marian Miller, the postpartum patient, still can't urinate. So, the doctor orders insertion of a Foley catheter. Do you know how to catheterize her?*

Gather the same equipment as you would for a straight catheterization procedure. However, instead of a Robinson catheter, use a No.14 French Foley catheter with a 5 cc balloon. The Foley catheter care kit includes a prefilled syringe and a urine drainage bag with drainage tubing attached. The catheter may be preattached to the drainage tubing.

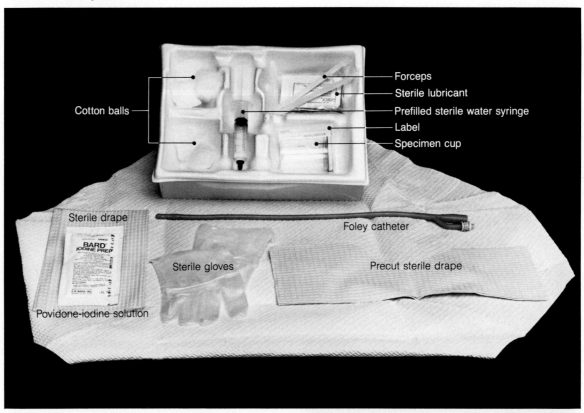

Cotton balls

Forceps

Sterile lubricant

Prefilled sterile water syringe

Label

Specimen cup

Sterile drape

Foley catheter

Sterile gloves

Precut sterile drape

Povidone-iodine solution

2 Explain the procedure to your patient. Review her chart carefully and make sure you have a doctor's order for Foley catheter insertion. Check the order to ascertain which size Foley should be used as well as any special catheter care the doctor has ordered. Read the doctor's progress notes to determine why Foley catheter insertion was needed and to see if any contraindications exist. For example, if the patient has a urethral fistula or tumor, contact the doctor before proceeding with catheterization.

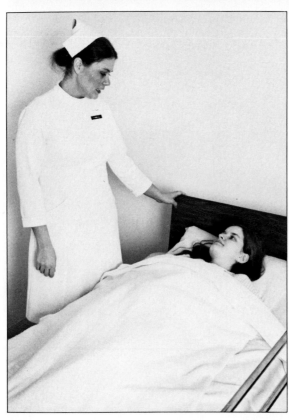

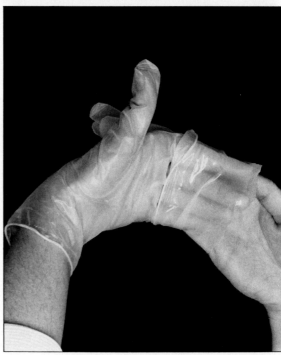

3 Place the patient in the lithotomy position. Open the catheter kit aseptically and put it between the patient's legs. Put on sterile gloves, as the nurse is doing here, and drape the patient, as on page 27.

4 You'll be following basically the same procedure as the one for straight catheterization, which was explained on pages 26 to 29. But, after you've put on sterile gloves, test the catheter balloon for leaks. Do this by attaching the water-filled syringe to the catheter's inflation port. (If your kit includes a syringe prefilled with jelly, be sure not to confuse it with the water-filled syringe.)

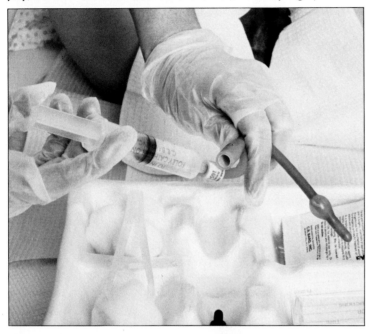

5 Now, clean the patient, as indicated on page 27.
Remember: The hand used to separate the labia is now contaminated. Proceed with catheter insertion.

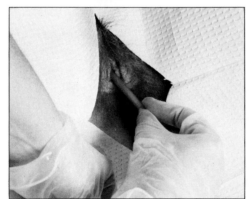

6 Now, obtain a urine specimen, according to the method outlined on page 29.
Note: If the catheter and drainage tubing are preconnected, don't disconnect them to take the specimen. Instead, take the specimen from the drain tube of the drainage bag.

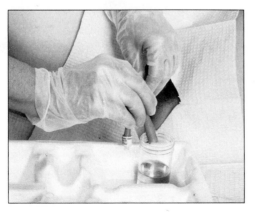

7 Now you're ready to inflate the balloon. First, pinch off the catheter with one hand. With the other hand (the one that's still sterile), advance the catheter an inch or two, so it's well into the bladder. This will provide enough space for balloon inflation.

Attach the prefilled syringe to the balloon port of the catheter. Inject all the water in the syringe, to inflate the balloon and keep the catheter in place.

Note: A 5 cc balloon requires 10 ml of water for complete inflation. A 10 cc balloon requires 15 ml. A 30 cc balloon, being less flexible, requires just 30 ml.

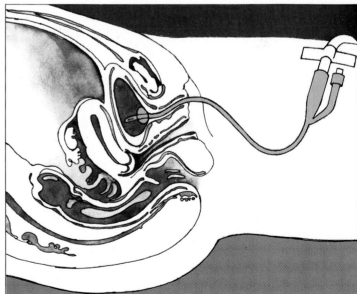

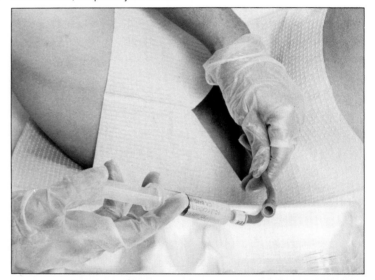

8 Proceed slowly when you're filling the balloon. If the patient expresses pain, the balloon may be in her urethra. Deflate the balloon immediately. Then, advance the catheter a little farther and reinflate. When you're sure that the balloon's well into your patient's bladder and completely inflated, gently pull on the catheter until you feel resistance. Resistance indicates that the balloon's positioned correctly, which ensures good drainage. Remove the syringe from the balloon port and check the port for leaks.

Indwelling catheterization

Inserting a Foley catheter into a female patient continued

9 Now, connect the catheter to the drainage tubing and begin collecting urine. *Important:* Never allow more than 700 ml of urine to drain from the bladder. This could cause the patient to go into shock or his bladder to invert. As soon as 700 ml urine drains, clamp the catheter.

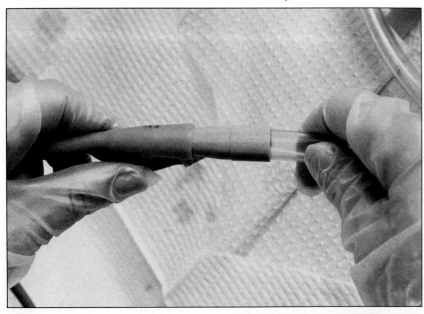

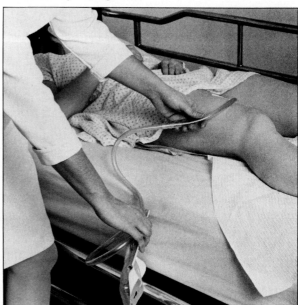

11 Position the drainage tubing over the patient's thigh or under her knee. Don't let it kink or loop. If the catheter kit has a clip, clip the tubing to the sheet so that it stays straight.

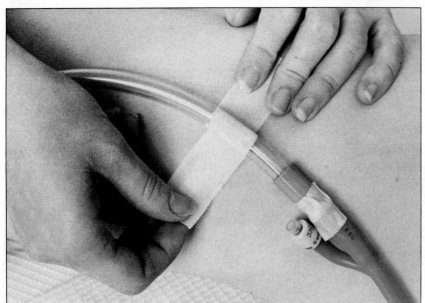

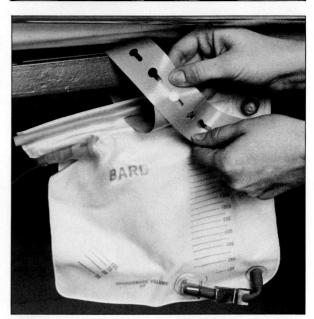

10 To avoid catheter pull on the bladder, secure the drainage tubing to the patient. To do this, first decide on which side of the bed you want to hang the drainage bag. Then, tape the tubing to the patient's inner thigh on that side, just below the perineum. If necessary, shave the area first. But don't ever apply adherents, such as benzoin, which will excoriate her skin. Use as little tape as possible, to avoid irritating the patient's skin, and make sure it's non-allergenic. Leave a small amount of slack in the catheter to minimize pulling caused by patient movement.
☛ *Nursing tip:* To make sure the catheter and drainage tubing stay securely connected, tape that junction to the patient's thigh, instead of taping the drainage tubing.

12 Use the fasteners in your kit to attach the drainage bag to the side of the bed. Be sure you attach the bag to the bed frame and not to a side rail. Otherwise, the bag may be raised above the patient's bladder. *Important:* Never place the drainage bag on the floor or it will become contaminated.

Examine and document the urine specimen the same way as for straight catheterization. On the patient's care plan, record your care, including any patient teaching you've done. Also, record how the patient tolerated catheterization.

Inserting a Foley catheter into a male patient

1 *How do you insert a Foley catheter into a male patient? Assemble the same equipment used for female Foley catheterization, detailed on page 36. But, follow a procedure similar to male straight catheterization.* Explain the procedure to your patient and review his chart carefully. Check the doctor's orders for Foley size and any special catheter care. Read the doctor's progress notes and contact him if any contraindications, such as bladder-neck obstruction, exist.

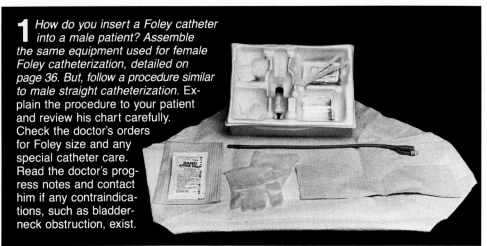

2 Position your patient flat on his back, as shown here. Drape and clean him, as indicated on pages 30-32. But, after you put on sterile gloves, test the catheter balloon, as you would do for female Foley catheterization (see page 37).

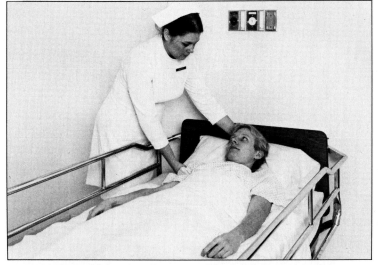

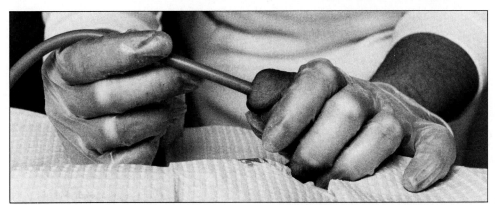

3 Now, proceed with catheter insertion. When urine begins to drain, obtain a specimen. *Note:* If the catheter and drainage tubing are preconnected, don't disconnect them to take the specimen. Instead, take the specimen from the drain tube of the drainage bag.

After obtaining the specimen, continue inserting the catheter up to the fork of the Y tube. Doing so ensures that the balloon's in the patient's bladder and not in his urethra. Now, inflate the balloon, following the instructions on page 37 for female Foley catheterization.

4 Connect the distal end of the catheter to the drainage tubing and allow urine to drain into the bag.
Remember: Never collect more then 700 ml urine at one time. (If 700 ml drains, clamp the tubing immediately.)

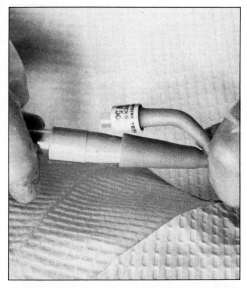

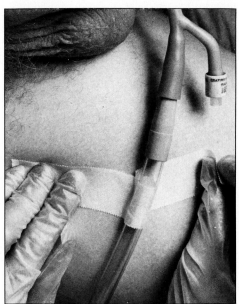

5 Decide on which side of the bed you want the drainage bag to hang. Then, keep the drainage tubing in place by taping it (not the catheter) to the patient's inner thigh on that side, opposite the base of the penis. If necessary, shave the area first. Use as little tape as possible, making sure it's nonallergenic, to avoid irritating the patient's skin. Finally, document the procedure and send the properly labeled urine specimen to the lab.

Indwelling catheterization

Caring for the patient with a Foley catheter

After you've aseptically inserted a Foley catheter, take these measures to help prevent urinary tract infection and to keep the catheter draining freely:
* Always wash your hands before and after touching the catheter, tubing, or bag.
* Check the catheter for proper drainage every time you have contact with the patient. At a minimum, make sure the catheter's checked once every 8 hours.
* Keep the drainage tubing/catheter junction closed, except to irrigate an obstructed catheter. When you must disconnect the tube from the catheter, use aseptic technique. (See the photostory beginning on page 46 for more details.)
* Don't allow the tubing to kink or loop, or it might block the urine flow, causing urine to reflux into the patient's bladder. As you know, urine reflux can cause bladder distention or infection.
* Keep the bag below bladder level to prevent urine reflux. (See the photostory on this page.)
* Never clamp the drainage tubing, unless you're obtaining a urine specimen or transferring your patient. Then, do it only briefly. Prolonged clamping causes urine to reflux into the bladder.
* Don't place the drainage bag on the floor or the bag may become contaminated.
* Empty the drainage bag at least once every 8 hours. Use aseptic technique when emptying the drainage bag (see the photostory on page 41.)
* Clean the patient's periurethral area, his perineum, and his anal area twice daily with soap and water. Pat dry with a towel. Wash the skin around the catheter, where it enters the meatus. Don't use antiseptic ointment on the periurethral site, because prolonged use can irritate the tissues. For the same reason, don't use lotions, creams, or soaps containing lotions. Inspect the skin in this area every 8 hours for signs of irritation.
* Check the catheter once every 8 hours to see if it needs changing. To determine this, study the transparent tubing; you may see incrustations in the lumen. If you can't *see* any deposits, try rolling the catheter between your fingers. A gritty feeling indicates that calcium deposits have formed. Either of these signs warrants a catheter change. Latex catheters usually need changing once every 7 to 10 days, but Silastic™ catheters may last as long as a month.
* Ensure adequate fluid intake to prevent pooling of residual urine. Pooled urine fosters bacterial growth.
* Give the patient ascorbic acid, as ordered by the doctor, to acidify his urine. Acidity inhibits bacterial growth.

Keeping a drainage bag below bladder level

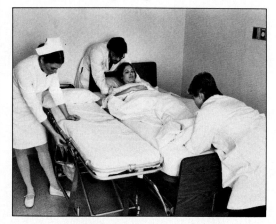

1 *Urine that's been collected in a drainage bag may have a high bacterial count. To prevent this urine from refluxing into your patient's bladder, keep the drainage bag below bladder level at all times.*

If you're transferring a patient from a bed to a stretcher, or from a stretcher to a surgical or X-ray table, have an extra person keep the bag below bladder level.

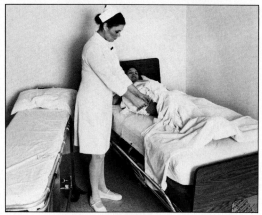

2 If you're working alone and you can't avoid raising the bag during the transfer, briefly clamp the tubing near the catheter-tubing junction just before you raise the bag. Then, as soon as possible, lower the bag below bladder level and unclamp the tubing.

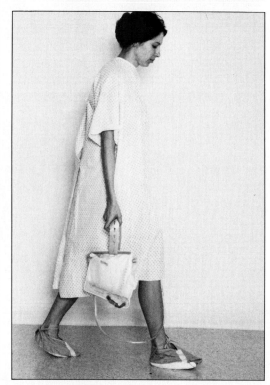

3 If the patient's ambulatory, have her carry her own drainage bag. Instruct her to keep it below bladder level at all times.

Emptying a drainage bag

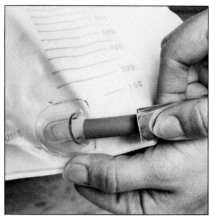

1 *Your patient's drainage bag must be emptied every 8 hours. When you do this, use aseptic technique. And, always remember to wash your hands before and after touching the bag.*

Now, let's discuss the procedure. First, remove the drain tube from its protective sleeve at the bottom of the bag. Be careful to avoid touching the end of the tube.

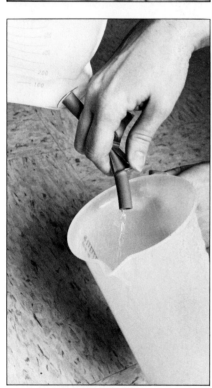

2 Next, unclamp the tube and allow it to drain into a graduated receptacle. Don't let the tube or your fingers touch the sides of the receptacle. Drain the bag completely. If you don't, old urine may foster bacteria growth in the bag.

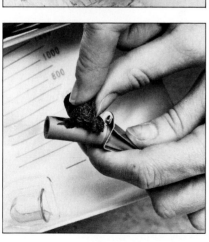
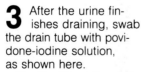

3 After the urine finishes draining, swab the drain tube with povidone-iodine solution, as shown here.

Finally, clamp the drain tube and return it to its sleeve on the drainage bag. Record on your patient's intake and output record the amount of urine drained. Empty the measuring receptacle and wash it with soap and water. Then, wash your hands.

Aspirating a urine specimen

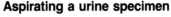

1 *Helen Ames, a 27-year-old housewife, had a Foley catheter inserted 2 days ago. Today, her doctor orders a urine specimen taken. You wonder, "Can I disconnect the catheter from the drainage tubing to take the specimen?" The answer is no. The only specimen you take from the open end of a Foley catheter is the specimen you take during the insertion procedure. In a closed system, once you connect the catheter to drainage tubing, you must keep the tubes connected. Otherwise, you risk introducing harmful bacteria into the urinary tract.*

To take a specimen, you must aspirate urine from the drainage tubing sampling port. To do this, you need a sterile 21G or 22G, 1½" needle, a 10 cc syringe, an alcohol swab, a label, and a sterile specimen container.

Sometimes urine is already flowing through the drainage tubing when you need a specimen, making it readily available. Usually, though, you have to clamp the drainage tubing and let some urine collect. If no urine's flowing, clamp the tubing 3" (7.6 cm) distal to the sampling port. Check for urine in 10 minutes. If enough has collected, withdraw the specimen. If insufficient urine has collected, check again in another 10 minutes.

Important: Never leave the tubing clamped for more than 10 minutes at a time without checking it. If you do, urine may pool in the bladder, causing infection.

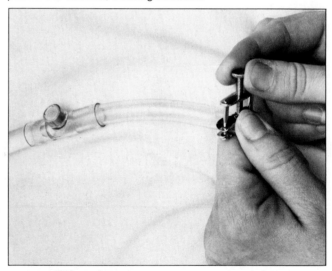

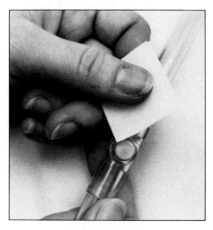

2 Before you aspirate the specimen, carefully clean the sampling port with an alcohol swab.

Indwelling catheterization

Aspirating a urine specimen continued

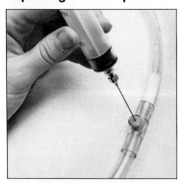

3 Attach the needle to the syringe. Then, uncap the needle on the syringe and insert it into the sampling port to withdraw the specimen.

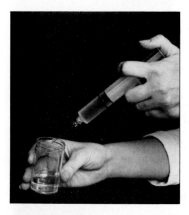

4 Transfer the urine from the syringe to a specimen container, and label the container. Immediately send the specimen to the lab.
Important: If for any reason you can't send the specimen right away, place it in the refrigerator or pack it in ice. Finally, add the amount of the urine specimen to the patient's intake/output record.

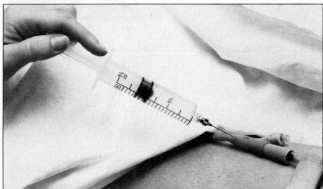

5 Suppose the drainage tubing you're using has no sampling port. If the catheter is rubber and self-sealing, you can aspirate the urine specimen from the distal end of the catheter. But, remember, this works only with rubber catheters. Silastic, silicone, or plastic catheters are not self-sealing.

To withdraw a urine sample this way, first clamp the drainage tubing 3″ from the catheter-tubing junction. Then, use antiseptic to clean the distal end of the catheter. Insert the needle at a 45° angle, as shown here. Inserting the needle at this angle ensures that the rubber self-seals. It also helps prevent puncturing the opposite wall of the catheter.

Important: Never draw urine from the shaft of the catheter; you might deflate the balloon.

Now, withdraw your specimen. Remove the needle, label the specimen, and send it to the lab. *Remember:* To ensure a fresh, sterile specimen, never collect a specimen from the drainage bag, except for a 24-hour urine sample.

Connecting a urine meter to a Foley catheter

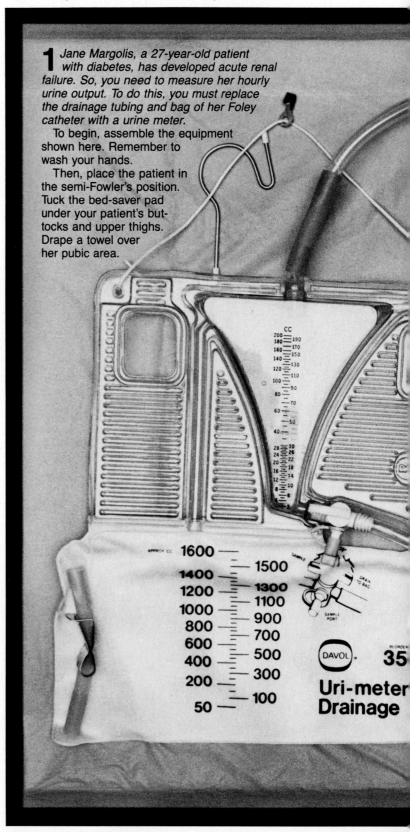

1 Jane Margolis, a 27-year-old patient with diabetes, has developed acute renal failure. So, you need to measure her hourly urine output. To do this, you must replace the drainage tubing and bag of her Foley catheter with a urine meter.

To begin, assemble the equipment shown here. Remember to wash your hands.

Then, place the patient in the semi-Fowler's position. Tuck the bed-saver pad under your patient's buttocks and upper thighs. Drape a towel over her pubic area.

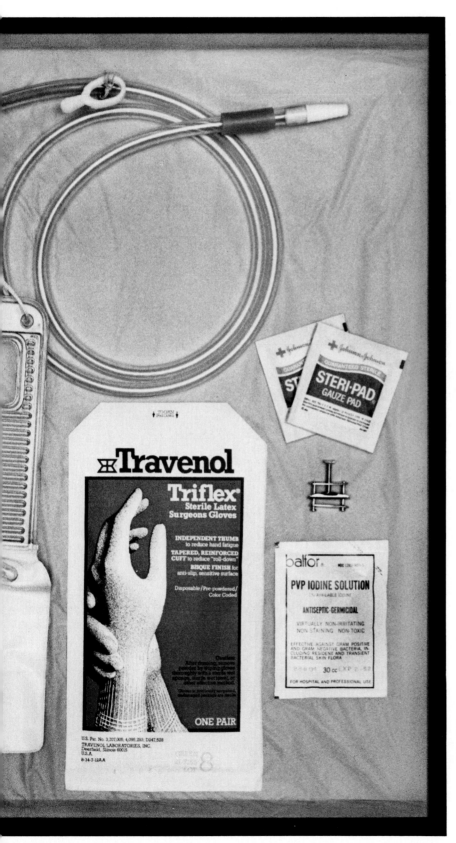

2 Clamp the Foley catheter. Then, straighten the drainage tubing to drain all urine into the drainage bag. Empty the drainage bag, using the strict aseptic technique described on page 41.

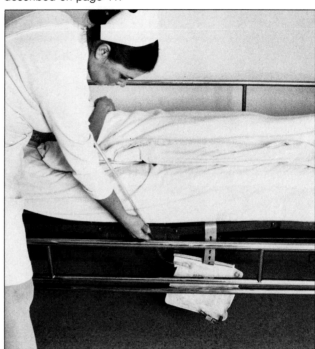

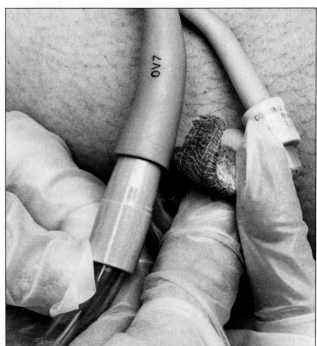

3 Open two sterile gauze-pad packets and moisten the pads with a small amount of povidone-iodine solution. Then, put on sterile gloves. Now, use the gauze pads to thoroughly clean the junction of the catheter and the drainage tubing.

Indwelling catheterization

Connecting a urine meter to a Foley catheter continued

4 Next, you'll disconnect the catheter from the drainage tubing.

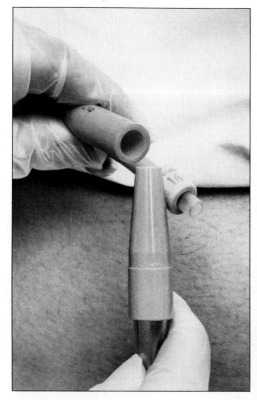

5 Holding the end of the catheter between two fingers of one hand, use that hand to pull off the cap of the urine-meter tubing. Don't touch the tip of the urine-meter tubing with your fingers or to the outside of the catheter.

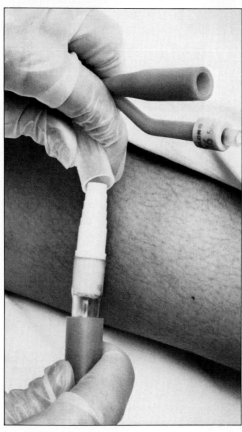

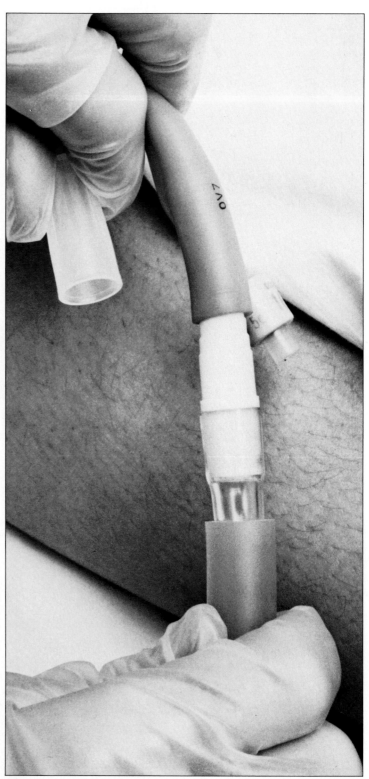

6 Now, connect the urine meter to the catheter. Then, unclamp the catheter. Arrange the urine-meter tubing so that it's as straight as possible, without kinks or loops. Doing this will help prevent obstruction and reflux of the urine.

7 Hang the urine meter on the side of the bed. Check the stopcock between the urine meter and the collection bag to make sure the stopcock's closed. Now, tape the tubing to the patient's leg. Discard the Foley drainage bag.

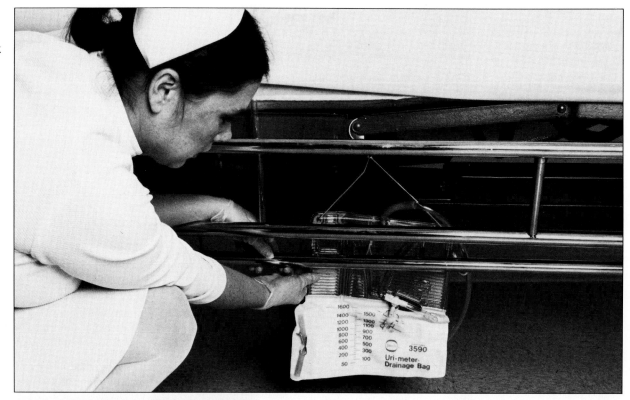

8 After the urine meter's been connected, check and empty it every hour. To do this, first record the amount of urine collected. Then, empty the contents of the meter into the drainage bag by turning a stopcock or by tilting the meter, depending on the model you're using. Turn the stopcock to the closed position. When that's accomplished, let urine collect in the meter again.

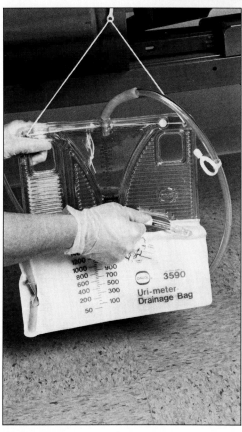

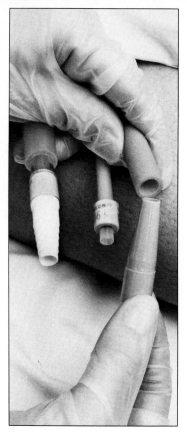

9 When the patient's hourly urine output returns to normal, and the doctor discontinues his order to record hourly output, disconnect the urine meter and replace it with a drainage bag and tubing.

To replace the meter with a drainage bag, repeat the steps taken to connect the urine meter. Assemble again the equipment pictured on pages 42 and 43. However, this time, substitute a sterile disposable drainage bag, with drainage tubing attached, for the urine meter.

Wash your hands. Then, position and drape the patient. Clamp the catheter. Drain urine into the drainage bag and empty the bag. Put on sterile gloves. Then, disconnect the urine meter and clean the end of the catheter, as before. Connect the catheter and the drainage tubing. Tape the drainage tubing to the patient's thigh. Then, arrange the tubing properly and hang the bag on the side of the bed.

Indwelling catheterization

Irrigating a Foley catheter: Initial steps

In the past, a nurse irrigated a catheter simply to wash out the patient's bladder or to instill prophylactic antibiotic drugs. But now we're aware that irrigation can irritate delicate tissues. Moreover, disconnecting tubing to instill antibiotics actually increases the risk of infection. That's why today you irrigate a catheter only when the catheter's obstructed, and then, only as a last resort.

If you check your patient's catheter and discover no urine's draining, first inspect the entire drainage system for obstructions, working back from the bag. Then, gently milk the catheter and drainage tubing to clear them of possible blockage. *Important:* Milk the catheter very gently. Forceful milking may dislodge the balloon.

If urine still fails to drain, make sure the patient's not dehydrated. If he's taking fluids orally, give him one or two glasses of water, but no more than 500 ml. If he's receiving fluids intravenously, increase the I.V. flow slightly. Then wait 30 minutes.

If you can't restore the urine flow by any of these methods, ask the doctor if you should irrigate. Never allow a Foley catheter to remain obstructed for more than 1 hour.

Irrigating a Foley catheter: The procedure

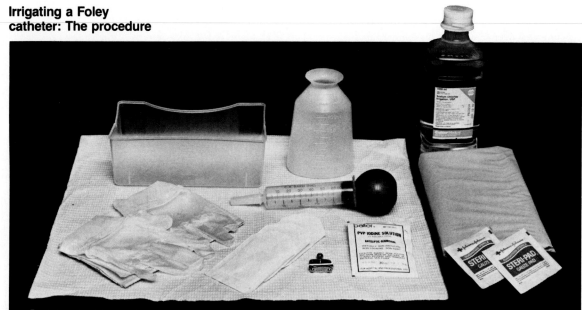

1 *John McNair, a 25-year-old telephone operator, is recovering from an appendectomy performed under spinal anesthesia. He's had a Foley catheter inserted for 24 hours. Suddenly, his urine flow diminishes dramatically. You determine that he's not dehydrated and that the drainage system is intact. So, suspecting a mucous or blood clot obstruction, you notify the doctor. He orders irrigation. In some cases, the doctor will* leave a standing order to irrigate as necessary.

To perform the irrigation using aseptic technique, assemble the equipment shown here: sterile irrigation set (includes solution container, bulb or piston syringe with rubber or plastic tip, gauze pads, povidone-iodine solution, drape, drainage-tube adapter bags, and drainage basin); irrigation solution (usually normal saline solution); bed-saver pad; Hoffman clamp; and sterile gloves.

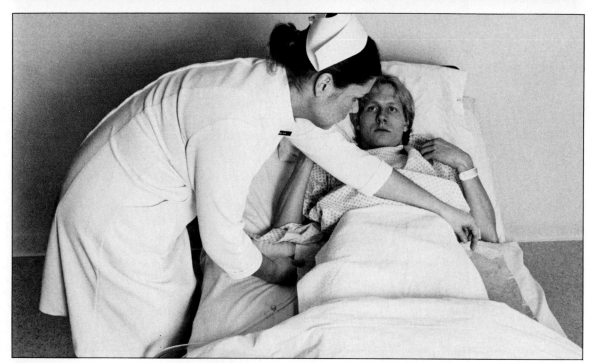

2 Now, explain to your patient the procedure and its purpose. Answer his questions before proceeding. Then, place him in a semi-Fowler's position, and tuck the bed-saver pad under his buttocks and upper thighs.

Nursing tip: To avoid exposing him unnecessarily, drape a towel or sheet over his pubic area, as shown here.

3 Next, wash your hands thoroughly. Unwrap the equipment, using aseptic technique. Then, open the bottle of normal saline solution, and pour 500 ml into the solution container. (Don't touch the inside of the container with the bottle; doing so contaminates the container.) Make sure the solution's at room temperature.

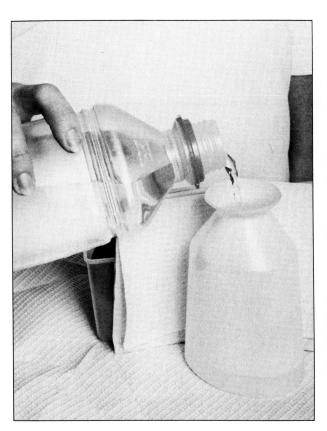

5 Next, clamp the Foley catheter below the Y-tube fork. Do this using a Hoffman clamp. Make sure you've secured the clamp as tightly as possible.

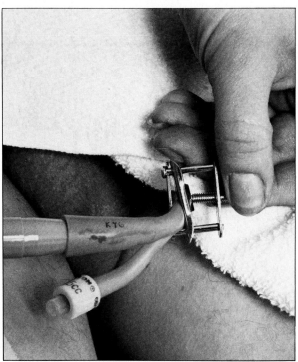

4 Use sterile gauze pads soaked in povidone-iodine solution to thoroughly clean the Foley catheter where it's connected to the drainage tubing.

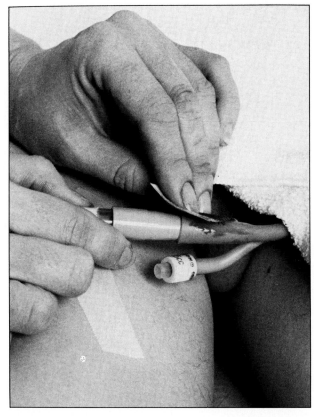

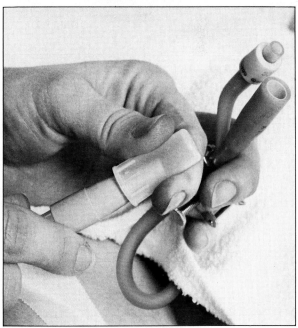

6 Carefully disconnect the tubing from the Foley catheter. Then, holding the catheter upright to keep it sterile, cap the drainage tubing with a sterile plastic tip or a paper adapter bag. Leave the capped tubing taped to the patient to keep the tubing from touching the floor.

Indwelling catheterization

Irrigating a Foley catheter: The procedure continued

7 Now, position your patient with his knees bent and his legs abducted. Place the sterile drainage basin under the Foley catheter, and make sure the basin's flat and secure on the bed. Put on the sterile gloves and draw about 50 ml of irrigating solution into the bulb syringe. Hold the catheter steady in one hand. Then, insert the tip of the syringe into the catheter, release the Hoffman clamp, and instill 50 ml irrigating solution into your patient's bladder.

Important: Take care not to instill the solution too forcefully. Never instill more than 50 ml at one time.

🔊 *Nursing tip:* With practice, you may be able to hold both the catheter and drainage tube upright in one hand while instilling the irrigating solution with the other hand (see inset).

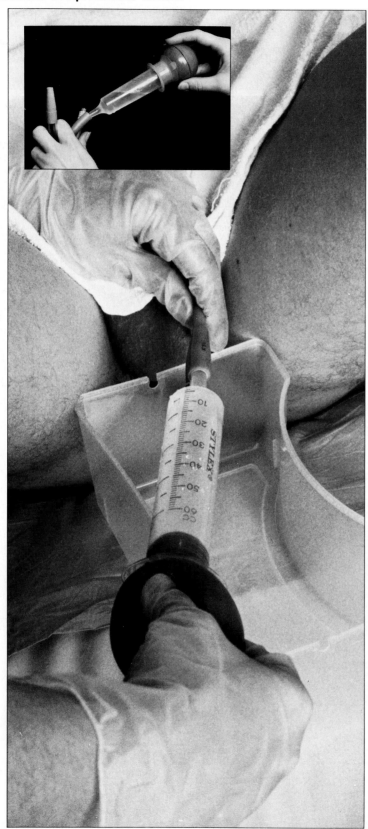

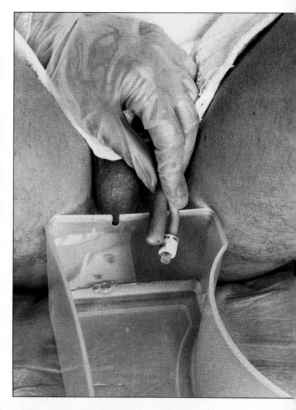

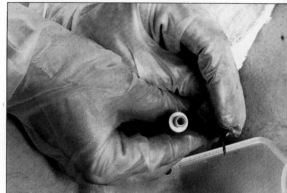

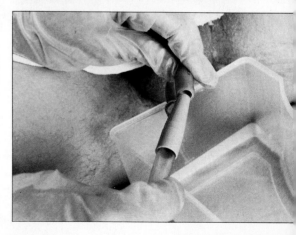

8 Now, remove the syringe and position the end of the catheter over the drainage basin. Collect the irrigation return in the basin and note its appearance. Is it cloudy, bloody, sedimented, or clear? Repeat the irrigation procedure until the returning fluid's clear.

Note: If fluid fails to return, stop instillation. An obstruction or air pocket may be present. Try gently rotating the catheter or turning the patient from side to side to clear the catheter. If fluid still won't drain, call the doctor.

9 Finally, clean the distal end of the Foley catheter and the end of the drainage tubing with povidone-iodine-soaked gauze pads.

10 Then, reconnect the catheter and tubing. Document the type and amount of irrigation solution used; the color and lucidity of the returning fluid; the presence of blood clots, if any; sediment, if any; and the patient's reaction to the procedure.

After irrigating, always discard any unused irrigating solution remaining in the container. Do not save the solution for future use.

Removing a Foley catheter

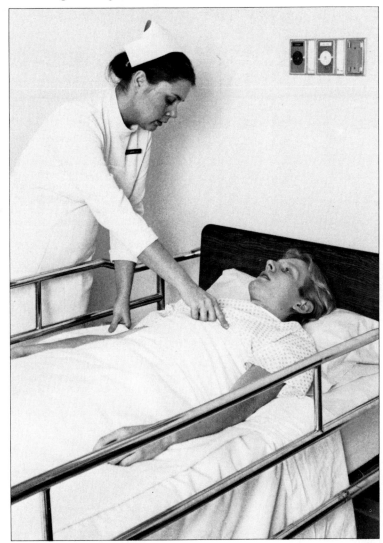

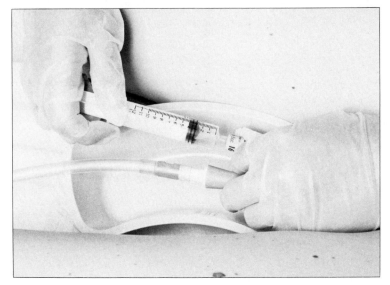

1 *You're about to remove a Foley catheter from a patient who's recovering well from surgery. Of course, you can't simply pull it out. The inflated balloon would severely damage his urethra. Instead, you must first deflate the balloon. To do this, don't snip off the inflation Y tube. That method's messy. Besides, if for some reason the balloon doesn't deflate, the doctor might want to use the Y tube to inject a dissolving solution. How should you deflate the balloon? By aspirating fluid from the inflation port of the Y tube.*

To prepare for this procedure, obtain clean examining gloves, an alcohol swab, a sterile needle, and a syringe big enough to hold the contents of the balloon.

2 First, put on the gloves. Then attach the needle to the syringe.
Note: If the Y-tube inflation port has a Luer tip, use a Luer-tip syringe.

Now, swab the inflation port. Then, insert the needle into it. Screw in the Luer-tip syringe, if you're using one. Withdraw the water from the balloon. This should deflate the balloon.

Indwelling catheterization

Removing a Foley catheter continued

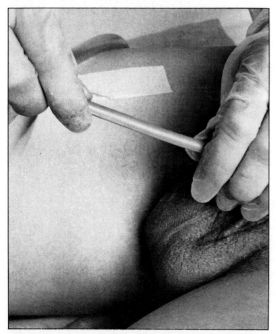

3 Now, you're ready to withdraw the catheter. Pinch the catheter near its tip, as shown here. Doing so will keep urine from draining into the urethra. With your free hand, gently withdraw the catheter and discard it.

If you can't withdraw the catheter easily, the balloon probably hasn't deflated. Don't pull on the catheter. Instead, call the doctor. He may inject 1 ml of lightweight mineral oil into the inflation port. The mineral oil will cause the balloon to break within 5 minutes to 1 hour. (You'll know the balloon has broken when the catheter feels loose in the urethra.)

When the balloon has broken, wash out the mineral oil and balloon fragments by irrigating the bladder. For irrigation instructions, see pages 47 and 48. Then, remove the catheter. To detect any fragments still remaining in the bladder, the doctor will order cystoscopy.

As an alternative to injecting mineral oil, the doctor may use ether to break the balloon. First, he'll fill the patient's bladder with 100 to 200 ml of sterile irrigating fluid. This will dilute the ether and cushion the bladder against balloon rupture. Then, he'll inject 1 to 3 ml ether into the balloon's inflation port. The ether will rupture the balloon within a few seconds. Prepare the patient for balloon rupture by telling him he'll feel a harmless popping sensation when it happens. To remove balloon fragments, the doctor will irrigate the bladder before withdrawing the catheter. Then, he'll order cystoscopy.

Give the patient a urinal or bedpan. Instruct him not to empty the collected urine until you're certain he's urinating normally. Continue an intake and output record for 24 hours after catheter removal.

Sending a patient home with a Foley catheter

The preceding photostories showed you how to care for a hospitalized patient who's had a Foley catheter inserted. But, sometimes the doctor sends a patient home with a Foley catheter in place. This patient must care for himself. Depending on his condition, the patient may use the Foley catheter for the rest of his life. Or, he may use it for only a few days. Either way, you'll have to teach him home care techniques.

Teaching your patient home care for long-term Foley catheter use
If your patient's a stroke victim, the doctor may send him home with a Foley catheter connected to a closed drainage system. A closed drainage system reduces the risk of infection that long-term catheter use entails.

Because your patient (or one member of his family) will be responsible for catheter care, provide thorough instruction before he leaves the hospital. To do this, give him a copy of the home care aid entitled "How to care for a Foley catheter connected to a closed drainage system," and a copy of the one entitled "How to empty the closed-system drainage bag," both on the opposite page.

Tell your patient that his Foley catheter's a rubber tube that drains his urine. Explain that a balloon on one end of the tube holds the tip inside his bladder. Then, show him where the catheter connects with the drainage tubing and the drainage bag; emphasize the importance of maintaining a closed system.

Teach him how to prevent infection by performing daily periurethral care, and stress the importance of using aseptic technique when emptying the drainage bag.

Discuss with your patient any fluid intake restrictions, and any medication he'll be taking. On his copy of the home care aid, fill in the blanks for fluid intake instructions.

Allow for the unexpected. Tell your patient to call the doctor if he experiences urine leakage around the catheter, or symptoms of urinary tract infection. If your patient already has a low-grade urinary tract infection, make sure he knows it, and warn him which signs and symptoms mean the infection's worsening.

If your hospital has an *informed consent form,* explain the form to your patient and have him sign it. When your patient signs the form, he accepts full responsibility for his Foley catheter management and affirms that he understands what you've taught him.

But, suppose your hospital has no such form. In this case, record in your nurses' notes the patient teaching you've done. Document your patient's statement that he fully understands what you've told him, and that he gives his consent to going home with the Foley catheter in place.

Finally, tell your patient when to return to the doctor to have his catheter replaced, or how to make arrangements to have a visiting nurse do this. In most cases, catheter replacement is needed every 3 to 4 weeks.

Teaching your patient home care for short-term Foley catheter use
If your patient's recovering from bladder or urethral surgery, he may be sent home with a Foley catheter in place for only a short period of time. Because infection's less likely to occur in such cases, he can use a leg bag during the day and a closed-system drainage bag only at night. The leg bag makes ambulation easier.

Remember, make sure your patient understands how to empty the leg bag without contaminating it, as well as how to change from the leg bag to the closed-system drainage bag at night. Instruct him in all points of daily catheter care. Then, give him a copy of the home care aid entitled "How to care for a Foley catheter connected to a leg bag," on page 52, and a copy of the one entitled "How to empty the closed-system drainage bag," on the opposite page. Also, obtain your patient's signature on an informed consent form, or document his consent in your nurses' notes.

Because your patient will have a Foley catheter for only a short time, be certain he has an appointment to return to his doctor for Foley catheter removal. Or, give him the phone number of the Visiting Nurses' Association, so he can make his own arrangements. *Warn him never to remove the catheter himself, under any circumstances. Doing so could cause severe injury.*

Patient teaching

Home care

How to care for a Foley catheter connected to a closed drainage system

Dear Patient:
You've had a Foley catheter inserted for your use at home. This catheter is a tube that will continually drain urine from your bladder, so you won't need to use a bedpan or toilet to urinate. A balloon on one end of the catheter holds it inside your bladder.

To care for your catheter, follow these guidelines:
• Never pull on your catheter, for any reason.
• Never disconnect the catheter from the drainage tubing. Any break in this connection will let harmful bacteria into the system.
• Maintain good drainage from the catheter by frequently checking the drainage tubing for kinks and loops. Also, keep the drainage bag below your bladder level, whether you're lying, sitting, or standing.
• Empty the drainage bag every 8 hours. To do this, follow the instructions on the home care aid the

nurse gives you.
• Use soap and water to wash the area around your catheter twice each day. Doing so will help keep the area from becoming irritated and infected. Also, wash your rectal area twice a day and after each bowel movement.
• Drink _____ 8 oz. cups of fluid each day.
• Take the medicine prescribed by your doctor, following all instructions on the label.
• Contact the doctor immediately if you have any problems, such as urine leakage around the catheter, pain and fullness in your abdomen, scanty urine flow, or blood or particles in your urine.
• Return to the doctor on the following date to have your catheter changed: _____
Don't ever try to remove the catheter yourself.

Home care

How to empty the closed-system drainage bag

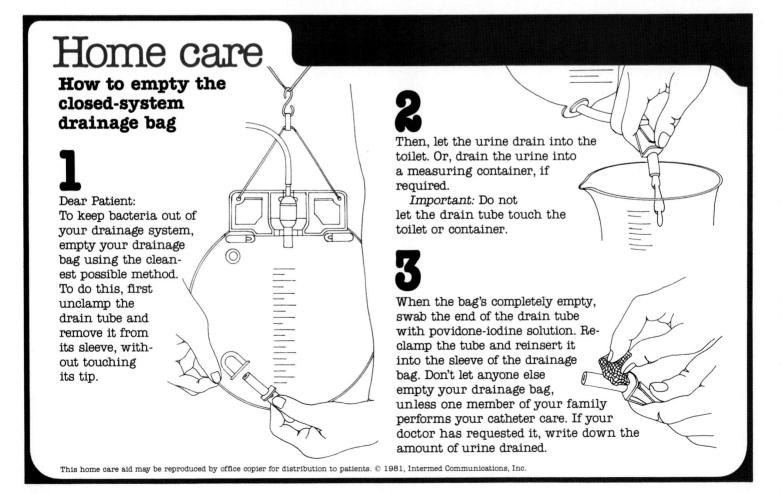

1

Dear Patient:
To keep bacteria out of your drainage system, empty your drainage bag using the cleanest possible method. To do this, first unclamp the drain tube and remove it from its sleeve, without touching its tip.

2

Then, let the urine drain into the toilet. Or, drain the urine into a measuring container, if required.
Important: Do not let the drain tube touch the toilet or container.

3

When the bag's completely empty, swab the end of the drain tube with povidone-iodine solution. Reclamp the tube and reinsert it into the sleeve of the drainage bag. Don't let anyone else empty your drainage bag, unless one member of your family performs your catheter care. If your doctor has requested it, write down the amount of urine drained.

Patient teaching

Home care

How to care for a Foley catheter connected to a leg bag

1

Dear Patient:
Your doctor feels you can return home, but your Foley catheter will have to stay in your bladder for the next few weeks. This rubber tube allows for continuous urine drainage, so you won't need to use a bedpan or toilet. A balloon on one end of the tube holds it inside your bladder.

As you can see, your Foley catheter's connected to drainage tubing, which leads to a drainage bag. During the day, you'll use a leg bag that straps around your thigh, as shown here. At night, you'll connect the Foley catheter to a closed-system (hospital-type) drainage bag. Because the leg bag is smaller than the closed-system bag, it allows you to move around more easily. However, you must empty it every 3 to 4 hours.

2

To empty the leg bag, first wash your hands. Then, remove the stopper and drain out all the urine. If requested by your doctor, drain the urine into a measuring container, so you can record the amount. Don't touch the drain port with your fingers or with the container.

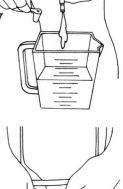

3

After the urine's drained completely, swab the drain port and the stopper with a povidone-iodine swab, as shown. Replace the stopper.

4

Before you go to bed, replace the leg bag with a closed-system drainage bag. Because the closed-system bag holds more urine, you won't have to worry about emptying the drainage bag during the night.

To replace the bag, first empty your leg bag. Now, clamp the catheter and swab the connection between the catheter and the leg bag with povidone-iodine, as shown. Then, disconnect the leg bag, and connect the closed-system drainage tubing and bag. Finally, unclamp the catheter.

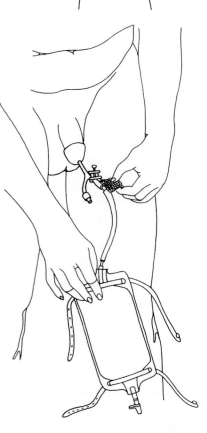

5

Now, decide which side of the bed you want the drainage bag to hang from. Tape the drainage tubing to your thigh on that side, using nonallergenic tape. Shave your skin in that area, if needed. Leave some slack in the line so that you won't pull on the catheter when you move your leg. If you're a man, tape the drainage tubing to the inner thigh, opposite the base of your penis, as shown above.

If you're a woman, tape the drainage tubing to the inner thigh below the vaginal area, as shown to the right.

After you've disconnected the leg bag, wash it in soap and water. Then, mix white vinegar and water in these proportions: 1¼ cups of vinegar to 2 quarts of water. Rinse the bag with this solution, to reduce urine odor.

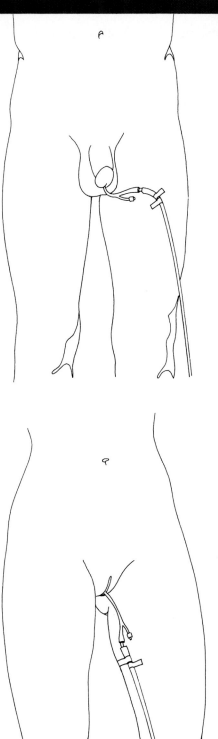

6

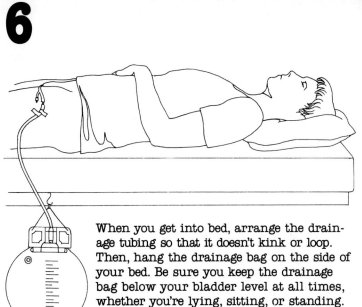

When you get into bed, arrange the drainage tubing so that it doesn't kink or loop. Then, hang the drainage bag on the side of your bed. Be sure you keep the drainage bag below your bladder level at all times, whether you're lying, sitting, or standing.

When you're ready to reconnect the leg bag in the morning, empty the closed-system bag. Then, repeat the steps you took when you connected the closed-system bag last night. But, this time, use the leg bag instead. Don't forget to empty the closed-system bag before you disconnect it. To learn how to do this, use the home care aid entitled "How to empty the closed-system drainage bag." When you've finished, wash out the bag with soap and water, and rinse it with the vinegar and water solution.

Note: You can reuse both types of drainage bags for up to one month.

To care for your Foley catheter properly, follow these guidelines:
• Use soap and water to wash the area around the catheter twice each day. This will help keep the area from becoming irritated or infected. (If you're a woman, wash your vaginal area as well.) Also, wash your rectal area at least twice a day and after each bowel movement.
• Never pull on your catheter, for any reason.
• Drink between _____ and _____ 8-oz. glasses of fluid each day.
• Take the medicine prescribed by your doctor, as instructed on the label.
• Contact the doctor immediately if you have any problems, such as urine leakage around the catheter, pain and fullness in your abdomen, scanty urine flow, or blood or particles in your urine.

Return to the doctor on the following date to have your catheter removed: _____

Don't try to remove the catheter yourself.

Catheterization self-care

You know that using a Foley catheter involves serious risks. But, do you feel you have no alternative? If so, you should know more about intermittent catheterization and urine collection without catheterization (external collection). You can perform these procedures instead of inserting a Foley catheter. Better yet, you can teach your patient to perform these procedures himself, with even less risk. Not only does self-care cut down on urinary tract infection, but it gives the patient a greater sense of independence.

To find out more about self-catheterization and external urine collection, read the following pages. We'll tell you all about:
• teaching a patient self-catheterization using sterile technique.
• teaching a patient self-catheterization using clean technique.
• teaching a patient how to perform external urine collection.

PATIENT TEACHING

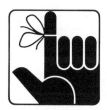

Teaching intermittent self-catheterization

If your patient has had a spinal cord injury and can no longer control his bladder, the doctor may order intermittent self-catheterization. With self-catheterization, the patient runs less risk of urinary tract infection than with indwelling (Foley) catheterization. The risk is less because the catheter isn't continually irritating the urethra and bladder, making them susceptible to bacterial invasion. Equally important, the patient has more control over his body so he feels more independent.

While your patient's in the hospital, he must learn to catheterize himself using sterile technique, because of possible nosocomial infection. Use the aids on pages 55 to 57 and 60 to 63 to teach your patient how. Make sure he understands why he must use strict sterile technique while in the hospital. At home, however, your patient can catheterize himself using clean technique. Use the aids on pages 58 to 59 and 64 to 65 to teach your patient the clean technique.

Note: When you teach your female patient self-catheterization, make a special effort to teach her which body parts are involved. Be sure she can locate her labia majora, labia minora, vagina, and meatus.

Obviously, the clean technique will be easier for your patient to master than the sterile technique. Fortunately, this advantage will make it easier for your patient to adhere to his required self-catheterization schedule. Make sure your patient understands how important it is to follow the schedule. Even if he has no soap and water handy, he must catheterize himself when his schedule requires.

Instruct your patient in these additional points about external urine collection. First, explain how he can regulate his fluid intake to prevent incontinence and still maintain a good hydration level. Second, urge him to take his medication regularly to increase urine retention and help prevent incontinence. (Consult the chart in the appendix for information about the seven most commonly prescribed bladder control medications.) Finally, tell him to avoid calcium- and phosphorus-rich foods, to reduce the chance of kidney stone formation.

Even though your patient's catheterizing himself intermittently, he may still experience incontinence. This incontinence will probably be a source of distress for him. Discuss the problem with the patient and his family, and remind family members that the patient needs emotional support. Also, help the patient and family develop a plan for managing incontinence. A visit from a public health nurse may be helpful in implementing the plan.

To control incontinence, the patient should wear some type of external collection device between catheterizations. To teach him how to apply and care for the device, see pages 68 and 69.

If the patient does have an incontinent episode, stress that he must perform adequate skin care. To perform proper care, the patient washes the skin with soap and water, and pats it dry with a towel. Then, he exposes the skin to air for as long as possible. Tell the patient how he can reduce urine odor by putting methylbenzethonium chloride (Diaparene®) or cornstarch on his skin.

Instruct the patient or his family to protect bedding and furniture by covering them with rubber or plastic sheets. They should cover the rubber or plastic with cloth.

When the patient's ready to be discharged, copy the clean-technique home care aid and complete the following: patient's catheterization schedule; prescribed fluid-intake, medication, and diet instructions; and record-keeping requirements (for example, for urine output). Discuss the aid with him to make sure he understands it. Then, give him the copy to take home.

Also, make sure he has enough supplies for at least 48 hours. Tell him where he can obtain additional supplies. You may contact a social service worker about keeping the patient well supplied.

Patient teaching

Self-care

How to catheterize yourself using sterile technique (for the female patient)

Dear Patient:
This aid will help you learn how to catheterize yourself. During your hospital stay, you must catheterize yourself using the cleanest possible method, because hospital germs are more dangerous than household germs. We call this method *sterile technique*. Practice sterile technique several times under your nurse's supervision. Soon, you'll be able to catheterize yourself easily. Here's how.

1 The nurse will get you this sterile equipment: a catheter care kit, including catheter, three cotton balls, forceps, sterile waterproof drape, povidone-iodine packet, water-soluble lubricant, container for draining urine, and two sterile gauze pads. She'll give you sterile gloves if your kit does not include them. She'll also give you a paper bag for discarding used equipment.

Use a mirror the first few times you catheterize yourself to help you locate your meatus. But, don't become dependent on the mirror. After a few catheterizations, you should no longer need it.

Before catheterizing yourself, try to urinate. To make this easier, press on your abdomen or stroke your inner thighs.

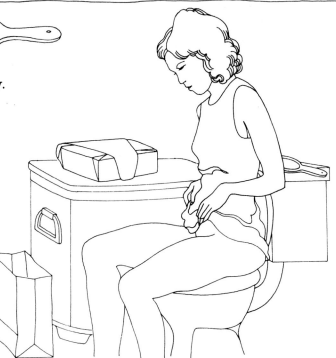

2 Wash your hands thoroughly. Now, position yourself correctly. For your first few catheterizations, you may find it convenient to sit on a bed, with your legs bent and your knees apart. After you become more skilled, you may sit on a toilet. Arrange your clothing so it's out of your way.

The nurse will get a small table for your equipment. Then, open the kit, making sure you don't touch its insides.

Patient teaching

Self-care

How to catheterize yourself using sterile technique continued

3 Now, put on one sterile glove, by grasping the folded edge of the cuff.

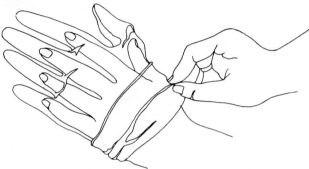

4 Then, place the fingers of your gloved hand in the cuff of the second glove and pull on the second glove, too.

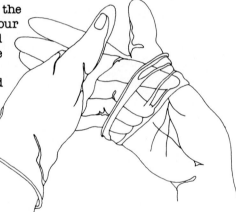

5 Now, lay down the sterile drape with the shiny, coated side down. Squirt sterile lubricant onto the drape. Then, open the povidone-iodine solution packet. Pour the povidone-iodine solution on the cotton balls.

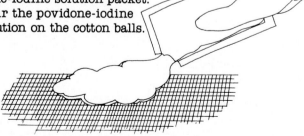

6 Now, use the gauze pads in your dominant hand to pick up the mirror. Be careful to touch only the gauze pads and not the mirror. Using the mirror, find your vaginal folds and urethral meatus. Hold the folds apart with your index and second finger. Identify the meatus. Remember, the hand you use to hold apart your vaginal folds is now contaminated. Don't touch anything sterile with it.

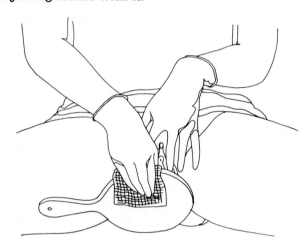

7 Now, clean your vaginal area. To do this, pick up the soaked cotton balls with the forceps. Clean the area between the folds with three downward strokes, using one cotton ball on the right downstroke, one on the left downstroke, and one down the center. Throw the cotton balls into the trash bag.

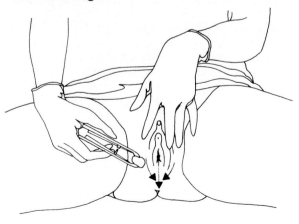

8 With your uncontaminated hand, pick up the catheter and roll the first 3″ of it in the lubricant.

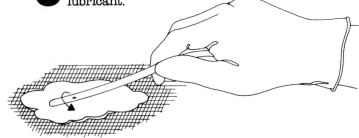

9 Holding your vaginal folds apart with your contaminated hand, use your other hand to grasp the catheter like a pencil or a dart. Insert it upward into the urethra. When urine begins to flow, gently push the catheter about 1″ farther. Then, allow all urine to drain from the bladder. Press down with your abdominal muscles and move the catheter in and out once or twice to help drain your bladder completely.

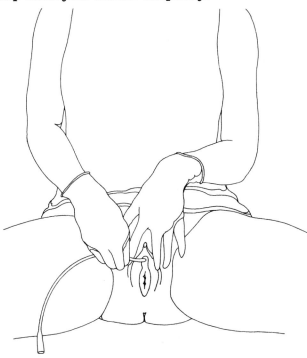

10 When the urine stops draining, pinch the catheter near its tip, to prevent urine from leaking into the urethra. Remove the catheter slowly. Tilt the tip upward as it comes out of the meatus, to avoid spilling urine on yourself. Then, throw the catheter into the trash bag. Dress yourself and dispose of the bag and used equipment.

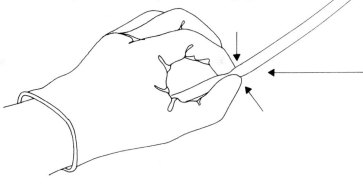

11 Finally, if your doctor requires it, write down the amount, color, and odor of the urine. Also, write down whether the urine's clear or cloudy. Note any particles or blood in the urine and tell your doctor about them at once. Let your doctor know immediately if the amount of urine increases or decreases; if you have difficulty catheterizing yourself; or if you experience pain or burning during catheterization.

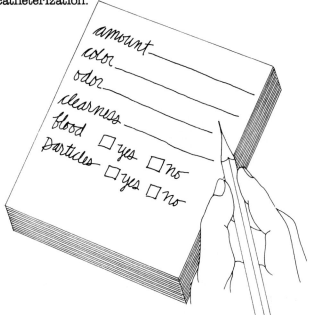

Patient teaching

Self-care

How to catheterize yourself using clean technique (for the female patient)

1 Dear Patient:
When you return home, you won't have to use sterile technique to catheterize yourself. Just take the few simple precautions outlined in this aid.

What's the most important point about a home self-catheterization program? To strictly follow your catheterization schedule. Otherwise, you'll retain urine, which can lead to an infection, a stretched bladder, or urine leakage. Never postpone catheterization, for any reason; for example, not having soap and water.

Cleanliness is very important, but on the rare occasion when you can't wash, your bladder's natural resistance to bacteria will protect you.

To catheterize yourself using clean technique, you'll need a rubber catheter, clean washcloth, soap and water, a small package of water-soluble lubricant, and a plastic bag for used catheters. Also, obtain a container for draining urine, if a toilet isn't available or you need to measure your urine. Make sure you have good lighting.

Before catheterizing yourself, try to urinate. Remember to wash your hands.

2 Now, separate your vaginal folds with one hand. Use downward strokes with the washcloth to wash the area thoroughly.

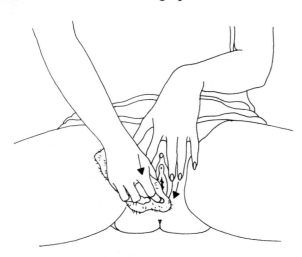

3 Lubricate the first 3" of the catheter.

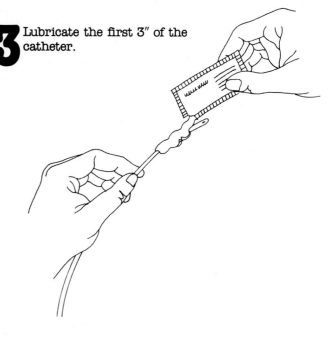

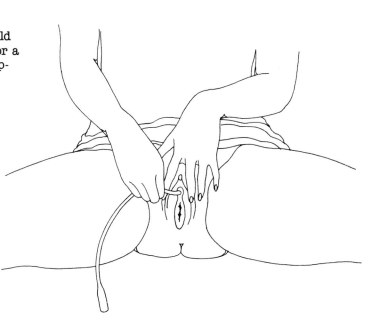

4 Now, you're ready for insertion. Hold the catheter as if it were a pencil or a dart, about ½ inch from its tip. Keeping the vaginal folds separated, slowly insert the lubricated catheter about 3″ into your urethra. Press down with your abdominal muscles to empty your bladder. Allow all urine to drain through the catheter. When the urine stops draining, remove the catheter slowly. Dress yourself, and wash the catheter in warm, soapy water. Then, rinse the catheter inside and out, and dry it with a clean towel. Place it in the plastic storage bag for used catheters.

Finally, if your doctor requires it, write down the information about your urine, as indicated below.

Buy a new supply of catheters each month or when the catheters become brittle. Use each catheter only once. When you've used all but the last catheter, boil the catheters for 20 minutes in a pan of water. Drain away the water and store the catheters in the pan or in a freshly laundered towel. Each time you use a catheter, be sure to put it in the plastic storage bag for used catheters, not back with the clean catheters.

Here are instructions tailored to your needs. Follow them carefully. Be sure you don't drink more than the amount indicated.

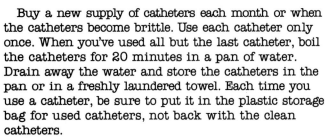

Catheterize yourself ____times a day at _____.

Each day, drink at least ____8-oz. glasses fluid, but no more than ____8-oz. glasses fluid.

The medication you're taking is:

_____

_____

This medication will help you control your bladder and prevent infection. Take all medication as directed.

Avoid calcium- and phosphorus-rich foods in your diet. This means that you shouldn't drink more than 1 glass of milk or eat more than ½ oz. of cheddar or Swiss cheese each day. If you eat other dairy prod-

ucts, such as other cheeses, ice cream, or yogurt, don't drink milk or eat hard cheese that day. And eat these other dairy products only in small amounts.

Also, eat only a small amount of the following foods: organ meats (for example, liver); shellfish; cereals; beans; dried fruits; and dark green vegetables (for example, kale, brussels sprouts, and okra). Limit eggs to one each day.

The doctor may want you to keep a daily record of the amount of liquid you drink and the amount of urine you excrete. Each time you drink any liquid, write down the amount. Each time you catheterize yourself, write down the information the doctor wants by following the form below.

Amount of urine _____.
This is (check one)
☐ increase   ☐ decrease   ☐ no change

Color _____

Odor _____

Clearness _____

Particles _____

Blood _____

Patient teaching

Self-care

How to catheterize yourself using sterile technique (for the male patient)

Dear Patient:

This aid will help you learn how to catheterize yourself. During your hospital stay, you must catheterize yourself using the cleanest possible method, because hospital germs are more dangerous than household germs. We call this method *sterile technique*. Practice sterile technique several times under your nurse's supervision. Soon, you'll be able to catheterize yourself easily. Here's how.

1 The nurse will get you this sterile equipment: a catheter care kit, including catheter, three cotton balls, forceps, sterile waterproof drape, povidone-iodine packet, container for draining urine, and water-soluble lubricant. She'll give you sterile gloves if your kit does not include them. She'll also give you a paper bag for discarding used equipment.

Before catheterizing yourself, try to urinate. To make this easier, press on your abdomen or stroke your inner thighs.

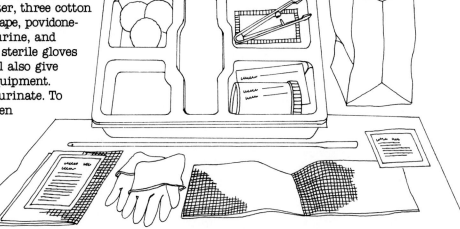

2 Wash your hands thoroughly. Sit on the toilet or on a chair for your first few catheterizations. Later, when you're more skilled, you can stand over the toilet. Arrange your clothing so it's out of your way.

The nurse will get a small table for your equipment. Or, if you're standing over the toilet, use the toilet-tank top.

Open the kit, without touching its insides.

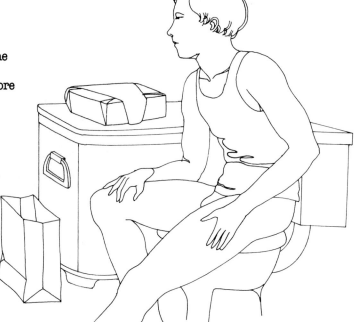

3 Now, put on one glove by grasping the folded edge of the cuff. [Inset] Then, place the fingers of your gloved hand in the cuff of the second glove and pull on the second glove, too. Then, position the drape shiny, coated side down and lay out your equipment.

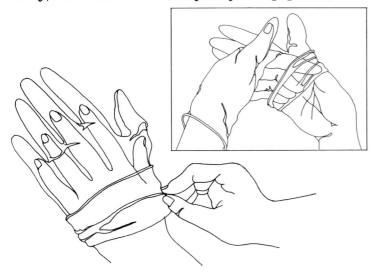

5 Now, you're ready to clean your penis with the saturated cotton balls. With your non-dominant hand, grasp the sides of your penis. *Note:* Don't use this hand for anything else during the procedure. If you're uncircumcised, pull back your foreskin with the same hand. Keep the foreskin pulled back for insertion.

With your dominant hand, use the forceps to pick up a cotton ball. Begin cleaning at the opening of your penis. Move outward in a spiral motion to the edge of the penis head. Discard the cotton ball into the paper bag and repeat this step until you've used all three cotton balls.

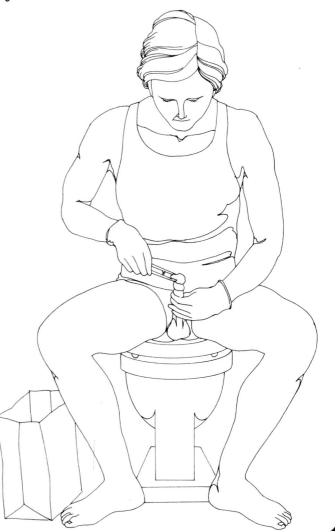

4 Next, squirt out the sterile lubricant onto the drape. Then, open the povidone-iodine solution packet. Pour the povidone-iodine on the cotton balls.

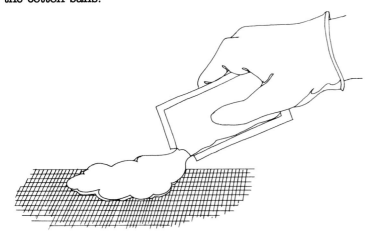

Patient teaching

Self-care

How to catheterize yourself using sterile technique (for the male patient) continued

6 With the same hand, pick up the catheter and roll the first 7" to 10" of it in the lubricant.

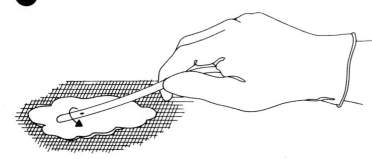

7 Now, using your nondominant hand, hold your penis at a right angle to your body, and prepare for catheter insertion.

8 Holding the catheter like a pencil or a dart, gently advance the catheter 7" to 10" into your urethra.

Never force the catheter. However, when the catheter is about halfway inserted, you may feel resistance. Applying firm but gentle pressure to the catheter will help relax tight muscles and permit the catheter to pass.

Note: If you're inserting a coudé-tipped Tiemann catheter, keep the tip pointed up at all times.

When the urine begins to flow, gently push the catheter 1 inch farther. Allow all urine to drain into the toilet or container; press down with your abdominal muscles to completely empty the bladder.

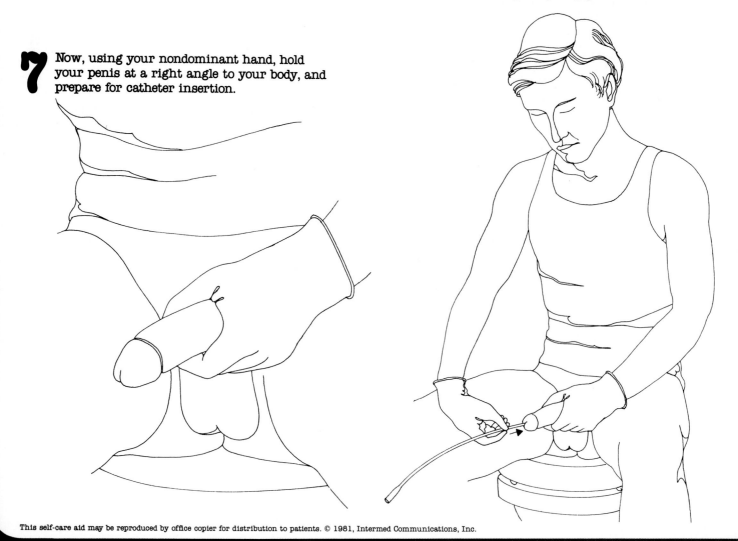

9 When the urine stops draining, pinch the catheter near its tip and remove it slowly. Tilt the tip upward as it comes out of the meatus, to avoid spilling urine on yourself. Discard the catheter in the paper bag. If you're uncircumcised, pull the foreskin forward again. Dress yourself and discard the paper bag and used equipment in the trash can.

10 Finally, if your doctor requires it, write down the amount, color, and odor of the urine. Also write down whether the urine's clear or cloudy. Note any particles or blood and tell your doctor about them at once. Also, let your doctor know immediately if the amount of urine increases or decreases, if you have difficulty catheterizing yourself, or if you experience pain or burning during catheterization.

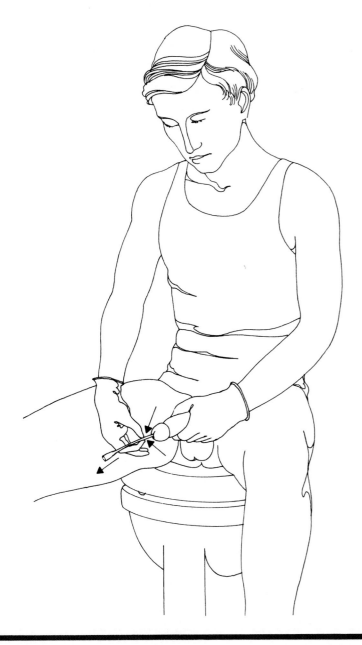

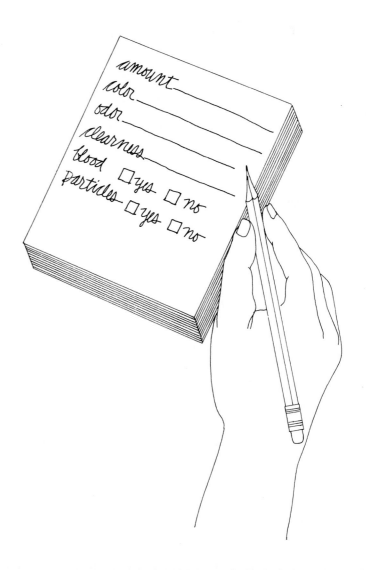

Patient teaching

Home care

How to catheterize yourself using clean technique (for the male patient)

1

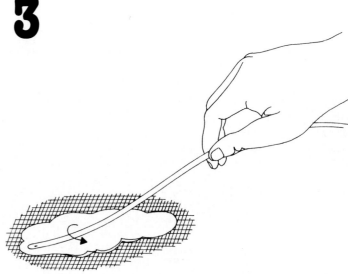

Dear Patient:
When you return home, you don't have to use sterile technique to catheterize yourself. Just take the few simple precautions outlined in this aid.

What's the most important point about a home self-catheterization program? To strictly follow your catheterization schedule. Otherwise, you'll retain urine, which can lead to an infection, a stretched bladder, or urine leakage. Never postpone catheterization, for any reason; for example, not having soap and water. Cleanliness is very important, but on the rare occasion when you can't wash, your bladder's natural resistance to bacteria will protect you.

To catheterize yourself using clean technique, you'll need: a rubber catheter, clean washcloths, soap and water, a small package of lubricant, a paper towel (not shown), and a plastic bag. Also, obtain a container for draining urine if a toilet isn't available or if you need to measure your urine.

Before catheterizing yourself, try to urinate. Now, arrange your clothing so it's not in your way. Remember to wash your hands.

2

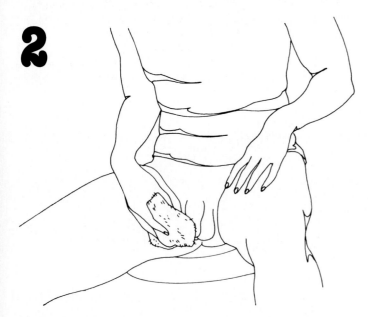

If you're uncircumcised, pull back your penis' foreskin and keep it back throughout the catheterization. Then, wash the end of your penis thoroughly with soap and water, as shown.

3

Squeeze some lubricant onto the paper towel and lubricate the first 7 to 10 inches of the catheter.

4

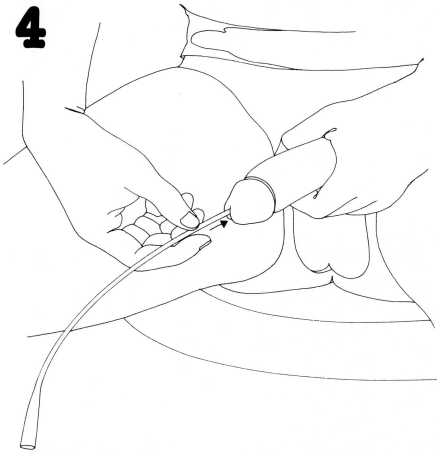

Then, hold your penis at a right angle to your body. Grasp the catheter as you would a pencil or dart, and slowly insert it 7 to 10 inches, until urine begins to flow. Then, gently push the catheter 1 inch farther. Allow all urine to drain into the toilet or container.

When urine stops draining, slowly remove the catheter. Pull your foreskin forward again. Dress yourself and wash the catheter in warm, soapy water. Then, rinse the catheter inside and out, and dry it with a clean towel. Place the catheter in the plastic bag.

Finally, if your doctor requires it, write down information about your urine, as explained to the right.

Buy a new supply of catheters each month, or when the catheters become brittle. Use each catheter only once. When you've used all but the last catheter, boil the catheters for 20 minutes in a pan of water. Drain away the water and store the catheters in the pan or in a freshly laundered towel. Each time you use a catheter, be sure to put it in your plastic storage bag for used catheters, not back with the clean catheters.

Here are instructions tailored for your needs. Follow them carefully. Be particularly cautious not to drink more than the amount indicated.

Catheterize yourself _____times a day at _____.

Each day, drink at least _____8-oz. glasses fluid, but no more than _____8 oz. glasses fluid.

The medication you're taking is:

_____

This medication will help you control your bladder and prevent infection. Take all medication as directed.

Avoid calcium- and phosphorus-rich foods in your diet. This means that you shouldn't drink more than 1 glass of milk or eat more than ½ oz. of cheddar or Swiss cheese each day. If you eat other dairy products, such as other cheeses, ice cream, or yogurt, don't drink the milk or eat the hard cheese that day. And, eat these other dairy products only in small amounts. Also, eat only a small amount of the following foods: organ meats (for example, liver), shellfish, cereals, beans, dried fruits, and dark green vegetables (for example, kale, brussels sprouts, and okra). Limit eggs to one each day.

The doctor may want you to keep a record of the amount of liquid you drink and the amount of urine you excrete. Each time you drink any liquid, write down the amount. Each time you catheterize yourself, write down the information listed in the form below.

Amount of urine _____
This is (check one)   ☐ no change
☐ increase   ☐ decrease
Color _____
Odor _____ Particles _____
Clearness _____ Blood _____

Catheterization self-care

Understanding external urine collection

You may think catheterization's the only way to manage incontinence. But many patients successfully use external urine collection. Do you know what this method entails? External collection for male patients usually involves applying a sheath or condom to the penis to collect urine. The sheath may have a drain port that can be connected to a leg bag for greater capacity. Female patients don't use sheaths; for them, external collection means wearing diapers, sanitary pads, or waterproof pants with disposable linings. Men also may opt for diapers or waterproof pants.

What are the benefits of external urine collection? The patient using external collection reduces his infection risks and eliminates the urethral trauma often caused by catheterization. And, in most cases, he'll be able to care for the collection system himself.

However, external collection does have its own risks: skin irritation, bladder infection, penile circulatory impairment, and disconnection of the collection system. You must take special precautions to avoid these problems.

Emptying or changing the collection device as often as necessary is an essential part of external collection care. The accompanying chart compares the different types of external collection devices; refer to it for changing and emptying schedules, as well as for other nursing considerations specific to each type.

Each time you change or empty a device, have the patient attempt to urinate. Then, carefully wash the penis (for a male patient) or the perineum (for a female patient) with mild soap and water. Dry the area gently, and, if possible, expose it to the air for a while before reapplying the device. Inspect the skin frequently for signs of irritation.

When you empty or change a reusable sheath, wash it in mild soap and water. Then, rinse the sheath with 15% white vinegar and water solution to deodorize it. Dust it with cornstarch to keep it supple.

Care for a leg bag in the same way. However, you don't need to dust the leg bag with cornstarch.

Nurses' guide to external urine collection devices

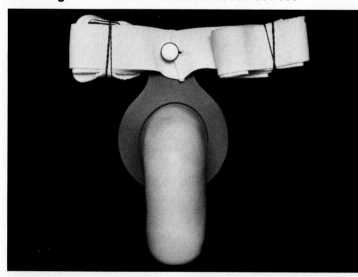

Dribbler sheath (Rusch)

Description
This rubber sheath straps around patient's hips. It has no drainage outlet.

Nursing considerations
• Use for mild incontinence (when patient urinates only a few milliliters at a time).
• Take special care to prevent skin irritation, because penis soaks in urine until sheath's emptied.
• Empty sheath every 2 to 3 hours, and perform recommended penile and sheath care.

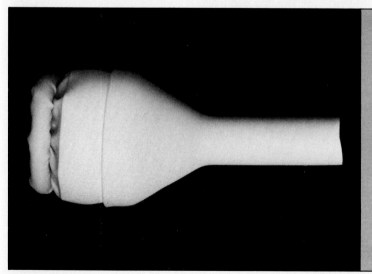

Single-layer urinary sheath (Chesebrough-Pond Uri-Drain® sheath)

Description
This close-fitting, latex sheath fastens closely around the base of penis. The sheath adheres to one side of double-sided adhesive tape that's wrapped around penis. Drain tube at bottom of sheath connects to a leg bag.

Nursing considerations
• Use for greater than mild incontinence.
• Perform penile care daily.
• Empty leg bag 3 or 4 times daily.

Double-layer urinary sheath (McGuire male urinal)

Description

This rubber sheath's held in place by attached athletic supporter. The sheath features an inner, tight-fitting layer that helps prevent urine leakage when patient's sitting or lying, and a loose-fitting outer layer for collecting and transferring urine. This design also protects penis from immersion in urine. The sheath's drainage outlet (with stopper) may be connected to leg bag.

Nursing considerations

• Use without leg bag for mild incontinence; use with leg bag for severe incontinence.
• Perform penile and sheath care daily.
• Hand wash athletic supporter, as necessary.
• Trim inner sheath with scissors to fit individual patient.
• Empty sheath every 2 to 3 hours, if used without leg bag. Empty bag 3 or 4 times each day, if used with leg bag.

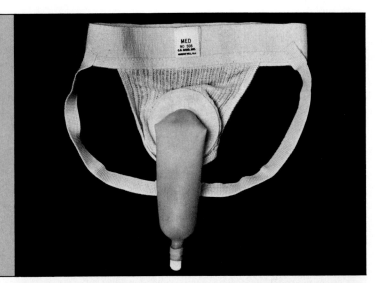

Condom catheter (Bard ® Disposable Uro® sheath)

Description

This soft, condomlike sheath fits closely around the penis. Sheath adheres to one side of double-sided adhesive tape that's wrapped around penis. Drain tube at bottom of sheath connects to leg bag.

Nursing considerations

• Use for greater than mild incontinence.
• Change catheter daily using a new one each time; do not reuse catheters.
• Perform penile care daily.
• Empty leg bag 3 or 4 times daily.
• Buy commercially made catheters, or make them yourself using condoms and rubber tubing, as described on pages 70 and 71.

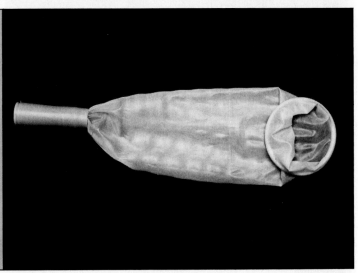

Diapers with waterproof coating, sanitary pads worn with waterproof pants, or waterproof pants with replaceable linings (Procter & Gamble Attends®)

Description

Diapers, pads, and replaceable linings are made of absorbent, disposable material. Diapers are plastic-coated on both sides to protect skin from urine irritation and to control seepage. Waterproof pants are made of rubber or plastic.

Nursing considerations

• Change frequently, as needed.
• Perform perineal care before completing change.

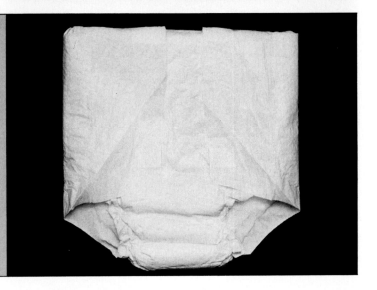

Catheterization self-care

Applying an external collection device

1 *You're intermittently catheterizing a quadriplegic patient. Because he's still having episodes of incontinence, he must wear an external collection device between catheterizations. The doctor orders a single-layer urinary sheath. Read the following photostory to find out how to apply it.*

Note: You can also use this same method to apply a condom catheter.

First, obtain a leg bag and a urinary sheath kit. This kit contains a sheath, Skin-Prep swab, and double-sided elastic adhesive.

Remember to wash your hands. Gently shave the base of the penis and its shaft, if necessary, to keep the adhesive from pulling on pubic hair.

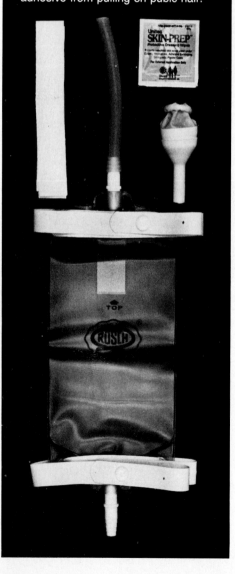

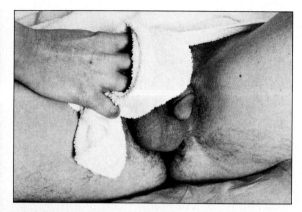

2 Then, wash your patient's penis and his perineal area with soap and water and rinse well. Dry the area thoroughly with a towel.

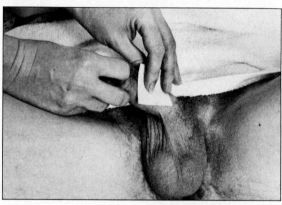

3 Now, prep the entire shaft of the penis with the Skin-Prep swab and allow the penis to dry.

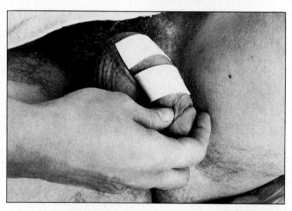

4 To tape the penis, first remove the covering from both sides of the double-sided elastic adhesive. Starting at the base of the penis, wind the tape in a spiral toward the glans penis. The edges of the spiral should not overlap. Never apply tape in a circle around the penis; doing so might cut off circulation. And don't stretch the elastic tape while you're applying it. If you do, the tape won't have enough slack to accommodate an erection.

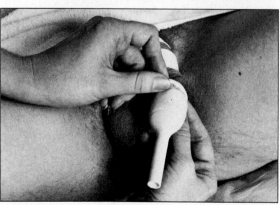

5 Remove the sheath from the kit. Make sure that the condomlike part of the sheath is rolled up to the edge of the molded sheath tip. Reroll it, if necessary.

Now, place the sheath on the end of the penis. Let the end of the sheath extend about ½" from the end of the penis. This gap will serve as a urine reservoir, so that the penis won't bathe in urine even if the urine backs up.

6 Next, unroll the sheath along the penis, gently stretching the penis as you do. When the sheath's fully unrolled, gently squeeze the length of the penis so that the sheath adheres to the adhesive tape.

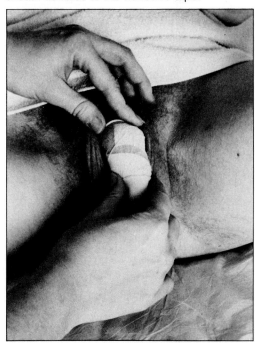

7 Connect the sheath to the leg bag, using extension tubing to join them together, if necessary.

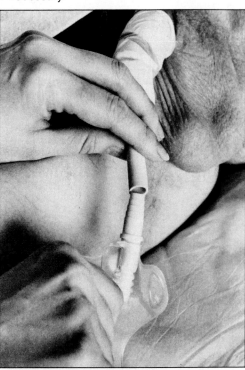

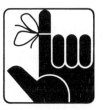

Teaching your patient condom catheter care

The doctor's encouraging your patient, who has an incompetent bladder, to use external collection rather than intermittent self-catheterization. You've put the condom catheter on your patient's penis the first few times, and you've shown him how to do that for himself. But since he's going home, he also needs to know how to care for his condom catheter and leg bag, and how to cut down on expenses by making his own catheters. Use the home care aid on the pages that follow to teach your patient all about condom catheter care. Give him a copy of the aid to take home.

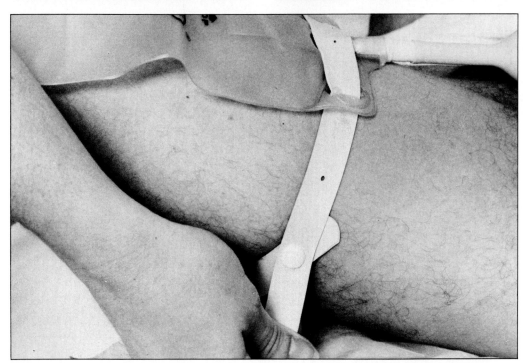

8 Strap the leg bag to the patient's thigh. Instruct your patient to maintain good gravity flow from the device by keeping his penis pointed downward, and by keeping the drainage tubing straight. Check sheath tightness in 15 minutes and again in 1 hour. If it's too tight, the sheath may impair circulation, causing tissue damage.

Patient teaching

Home care

How to make and care for a condom catheter

Dear Patient:

Now that you're going home, you'll be responsible for your condom catheter. For good home care, you must guard against skin irritation, bladder infection, impaired circulation in the penis, and disconnection of the collection system.

Do this by replacing your catheter with a new one once a day and by washing your penis carefully each time you change the catheter.

When you put on a condom catheter, be careful to apply the tape in spiral fashion, rather than in constricting circles. Make sure that the end of the catheter and drainage tubing stay straight. Twisted tubing may block urine flow. If urine backs up, it could disconnect the condom from the bag.

Although you can't reuse a catheter, you may reuse your leg bag for as long as 1 month. Empty the leg bag every 3 to 4 hours. Wash it twice daily with soap and water, and rinse it with a 15% vinegar and water solution.

Because you'll need a new catheter each day, you may find it economical to make your own, using a condom and drainage tubing. To do so, assemble a 5″ piece of ⅜″-diameter latex tubing, a condom, and scissors. Obtain condoms at any pharmacy. The tubing's available at medical-surgical supply stores.

1

Cut two ⅛″ bands from the end of the tubing.

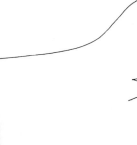

2

Place one of these bands around the tubing ½″ from the end.

3

Snip off the tip of the condom. Put the condom over the end of the tubing, with its rolled edge facing inward.

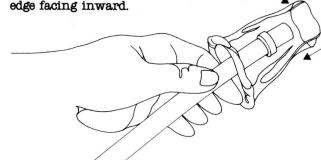

4

Now, take the second band and fit it over the condom on the tubing, close to the first band, as shown here.

5

Invert the condom so it extends from the end of the tubing.

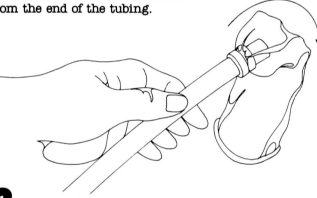

6

Pull the first band over the second. The bands are now about ¼″ away from the end of the tubing.

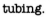

7

The catheter's now ready for use. Apply it the same way you applied the brand-name condom catheter in the hospital. If necessary, use extension tubing to connect the catheter to the leg bag. Strap the leg bag to your leg.

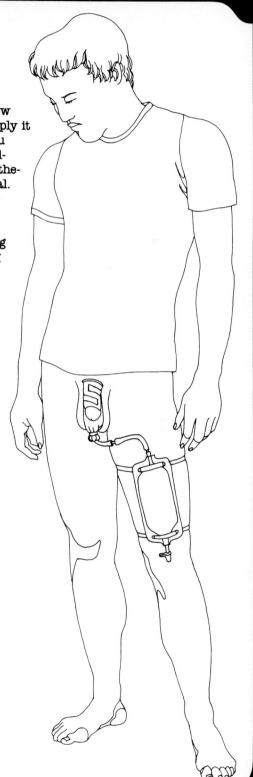

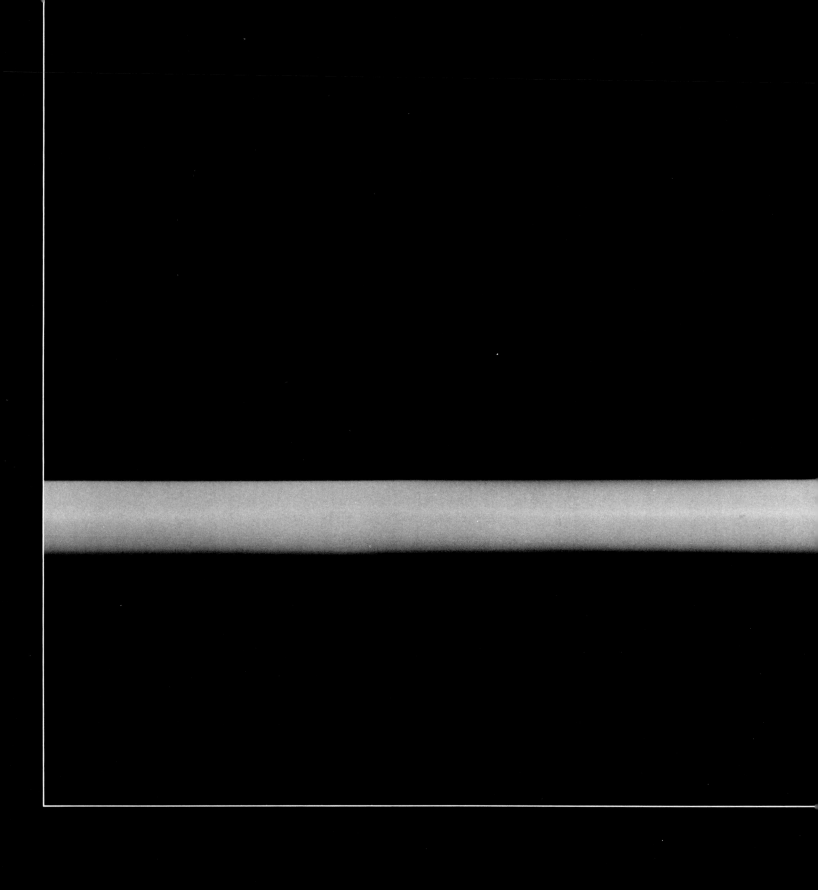

Caring for the Urologic Surgery Patient

Surgical care

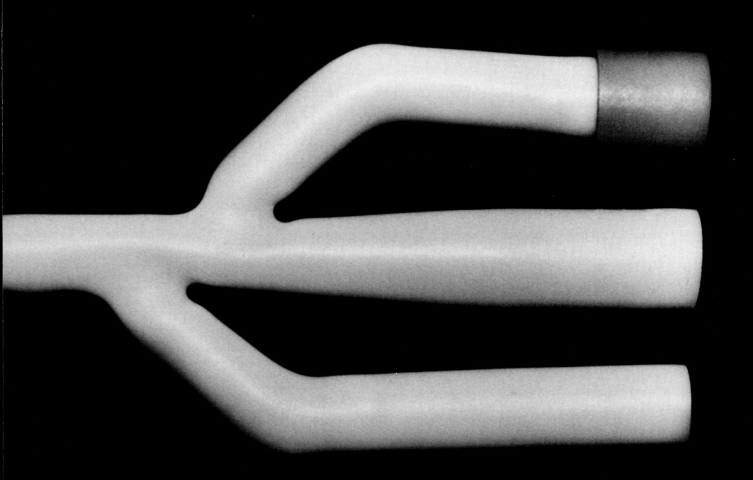

Surgical care

Caring efficiently for the urologic surgery patient requires diverse skills. To perform all aspects of surgical care, you'll have to know how to:
• prepare your patient for urologic surgery.
• differentiate between drainage tubes.
• apply a drainage tube dressing.
• irrigate a drainage tube.
• recognize signs of fluid and electrolyte imbalance, hemorrhage, and infection.
• care for the male patient with a penile implant.
• prepare your patient to care for himself.
   Sound challenging? Of course it is. But, by reading the pages that follow, you can make these tasks easier.

PATIENT PREPARATION

Preparing a patient for urinary tract surgery

What are your responsibilities in preoperative care? They are to prepare your patient so well that he undergoes as little psychologic trauma and physical complications as possible.

Start preop care as soon as the doctor's told your patient that surgery's necessary. Learn all you can about the surgery and the postop care involved. Find out how he'll return from the operating room. For example, what types of drainage tubes will he have? (Use the surgery summaries to the right as your guide.) How much discomfort can he expect? Also, remember to teach your patient any range-of-motion (ROM), deep breathing, or coughing exercises he may have to do after surgery.

Consider your patient's emotional state. Most likely, he'll be very anxious. Encourage him to express his fears. Perhaps some of them are unfounded and you can clear them up. As for his legitimate fears, allay them by emphasizing the positive aspects of the surgery; for example, how it will help prevent further complications, or how it will relieve his discomfort.

Some lower urinary tract surgery will leave the patient sexually impotent. Depending on your hospital's policy, the doctor will discuss this with the patient either before or after the surgery. Suggest postop sexual counseling for the patient, if appropriate.

The doctor may order dietary changes to strengthen the patient for surgery. This may include increasing the patient's intake of protein, vitamin C, and vitamin K.

The doctor may also order some of the diagnostic tests discussed on pages 20 and 21. If he does, prepare the patient for them using the guidelines detailed there. Because he'll also need a blood coagulation profile, and typing and crossmatching, make sure a blood specimen is drawn and sent to the lab.

Depending on your hospital's policy, you or the doctor must have the patient sign a surgical consent form. If he's having a vasectomy or an orchiectomy, he must also sign a consent form for sterilization.

Finally, the night before surgery, follow the doctor's orders for shaving and prepping the patient's groin, abdomen, or flank for surgery. You may also be instructed to give the patient an enema and strain his urine (if surgery's for calculi removal).

Learning about urinary tract surgery

Your patient faces urinary tract surgery. Do you know what kind? If you understand the surgery's purpose and procedure, you'll be better able to deal with your patient's specific needs. This chart is designed to familiarize you with all the basic urinary tract surgeries presently being performed. You'll find pre- and postop care considerations fully detailed in the pages that follow.

Urethra

Urethroplasty (to repair the urethra). The doctor will work internally to reconstruct the damaged urethra. He'll insert an indwelling urethral catheter to stent the urethra and facilitate healing.

Urethrotomy (to remove urethral strictures). The doctor will use a urethroscope or urethrotome to make an internal incision in the urethra and excise any strictures. He'll leave an indwelling urethral catheter in place for irrigation.

Prostate

Transurethral resection [TUR] (to remove prostatic tissue obstructing the urethra). The doctor will use a resectoscope that features an electrically charged wire loop to trim or chip away the invading prostatic tissue from the walls of the urethra. He'll leave an indwelling urethral catheter in place.

Suprapubic prostatectomy (to remove prostatic tissue obstructing urinary flow). The doctor will make an incision above the pubis and in the bladder wall to expose the prostate. He'll shell the obstructing prostatic tissue out of its bed with his finger. He may place a pack in the prostatic fossa and leave it there, along with a Penrose drain, for a day or two. He'll also insert an indwelling urethral catheter and, perhaps, a suprapubic catheter, to permit irrigation and ensure patency.

Retropubic prostatectomy (to remove prostatic tissue obstructing the urethra). The doctor will make a suprapubic incision and approach the prostate from between the bladder and the pubic arch. He'll make another incision in the prostatic capsule and remove the obstructing tissue. Bleeding vessels are cauterized or sutured and an indwelling urethral catheter and Penrose drain are put in place for drainage.

Radical perineal prostatectomy (to remove the entire prostate gland). The doctor will make an incision in the perineum and remove the entire prostate and seminal vesicles. Then, he'll suture the bladder to the urethra and close the incision, leaving an indwelling urethral catheter and Penrose drain in place.

Bladder

Cystolithectomy (to remove calculi from the bladder). The doctor will make a suprapubic incision into the bladder. He'll remove the calculi and then suture the bladder and the external incision closed, leaving a Penrose drain and a suprapubic catheter in place.

Segmental cystectomy (to remove tumorous bladder tissues). The doctor will make a suprapubic incision and open the bladder at a point away from the tumor. He'll remove the tumor, the attached fat, and the perineum with a 1¼" (3.2 cm) margin of healthy tissue. He'll close the wound, leaving a Penrose drain and a suprapubic catheter in place.

Simple cystectomy (to remove the bladder). The doctor will make a vertical or transverse incision in the abdomen and separate the bladder's posterior and lateral connective tissue. Then, he'll open the bladder near its neck and remove the bladder walls

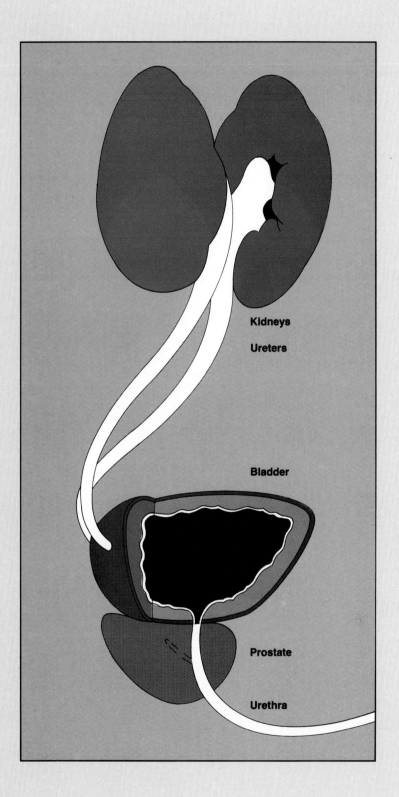

Kidneys

Ureters

Bladder

Prostate

Urethra

and surrounding tissue. He'll suture the bladder neck closed and bring the ureters to the skin to form an ostomy.

Ureters

Ureterolithotomy (to remove calculi from the ureter). The doctor will make either a suprapubic or a flank incision, depending on calculus placement, to expose the ureter. He'll slit the ureter to expose the calculus and remove it. Then, he'll suture the ureter and the cutaneous incision closed, leaving a Penrose drain and a suprapubic or flank catheter in place.

Ileal conduit (to permanently divert urine from the lower urinary tract). The doctor will make a suprapubic incision, excise a small portion of the ileum, and anastomose the remaining ileum to preserve intestinal integrity. He'll dissect the ureters from the bladder and anastomose them to the ileum segment. He'll suture closed one end of the ileum segment and bring the other end through the abdominal wall to form a stoma.

Cutaneous ureterostomy (to permanently divert urine from the lower urinary tract). The doctor will make a suprapubic incision. He'll dissect both of the ureters from the bladder. Then, he'll bring them together and through the abdominal wall, to form one stoma.

Continent vesicostomy (to divert urine from the urethra). The doctor will make a suprapubic incision, excise part of the bladder wall, and form a tube with the tissue without disconnecting it entirely from the bladder. Then he'll bring the constructed tube through the abdominal wall to form a stoma. The urethra is sutured closed.

Kidneys

Pyelolithotomy (to remove calculi from the renal pelvis or through the pelvis). The doctor will make a flank incision to expose the pelvis. Then, he'll make an incision in the pelvis and remove calculi or use the incision to enter the kidney and remove calculi there. He'll suture the pelvis and the cutaneous incision closed, leaving a flank catheter and a Penrose drain in place.

Nephrostomy (to divert urine from the ureters and the lower urinary tract in an emergency). The doctor will make a flank incision and expose the upper urinary tract. The kidney pole and pelvis are retracted and the pelvis is dissected. He'll feed a catheter into the kidney, and suture the other end externally at the patient's flank.

Nephrolithotomy (to remove large calculus from the kidney). The doctor will make a flank incision and expose the kidney. He'll isolate the renal artery (for later occlusion) and mobilize the kidney for optimal access. He'll inject mannitol into the patient's bloodstream to protect the kidney when the blood supply's occluded. After waiting 10 minutes, he'll clamp the renal artery, place a dam around the kidney and surround it with iced saline solution slush. Then he'll make an incision into the kidney (depending on where the calculus is) and remove the calculus. He'll suture the kidney and the flank incision closed, leaving a Penrose drain in place.

Nephrectomy (to remove one or both kidneys). The doctor will make a flank incision and expose the kidney. He'll mobilize the kidney and free it of fat and adhesions. Then, he'll free the lower pole, find the ureter, and free its upper third. The ureter is then doubly clamped. He'll cut between the clamps and ligate the ends. Then, he'll free and doubly clamp the vascular pedicle. Finally, he'll remove the kidney distal to the clamps, leaving a flank catheter and a Penrose drain in place.

Surgical care

Tube terminology

The patient who's had urinary tract surgery will return to your care with one or several drainage tubes in place. Your management of these tubes doesn't depend on what catheter the doctor inserted. Instead, it depends on *where* the catheter's inserted. Doctors usually refer to a catheter by its location. For example, a catheter inserted in the kidney is a nephrostomy tube, a catheter inserted in the renal pelvis is a pyelostomy tube, and a catheter inserted in the ureter is a ureterostomy tube. Because each of these tubes is inserted through an incision in the patient's flank, and managed accordingly, we'll refer to them in this book as flank tubes. A catheter inserted in the bladder above the symphysis pubis is often called a cystostomy tube. But, because it's inserted through a suprapubic incision, we'll refer to it as a suprapubic tube. And, as we've done before, we'll call the catheter inserted in the urethra a urethral catheter.

Differentiating between drainage tubes

During urinary tract surgery, the doctor may insert a Foley, de Pezzer, or Malecot catheter. He'll do this to divert urine from the surgical site, provide continuous drainage, and provide intermittent or continuous bladder irrigation. (Usually, the doctor will also insert a Penrose drain at the incision site for wound drainage.) Which catheter will he choose to insert? That depends in part on the purpose and in part on the doctor's preferences. This chart details how these catheters differ.

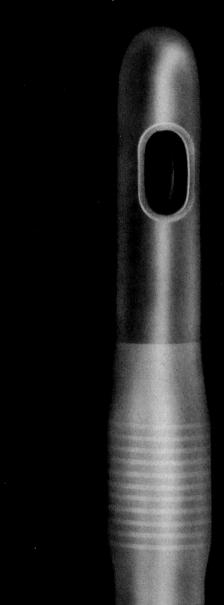

Foley
A double- or triple-lumen straight catheter with an inflatable balloon and a rounded tip. The double-lumen catheter also comes with a coudé tip.

Use
• To provide continuous or intermittent bladder irrigation as a urethral catheter
• To provide for bladder drainage and act as a stent as a urethral catheter
• To provide for bladder drainage as a suprapubic catheter

Special considerations
• Most commonly used for urethral catheterization

de Pezzer (mushroom)
A single-lumen straight or angulated catheter with a mushroom-shaped tip. The tip may have two or more holes in it.

Use
• To provide for bladder drainage as a suprapubic tube
• To provide for kidney drainage as a flank tube

Special considerations
• Must be inserted with the aid of a stylet, which temporarily collapses the mushroom tip.
• Usually sutured in place
• Not inserted into the urethra

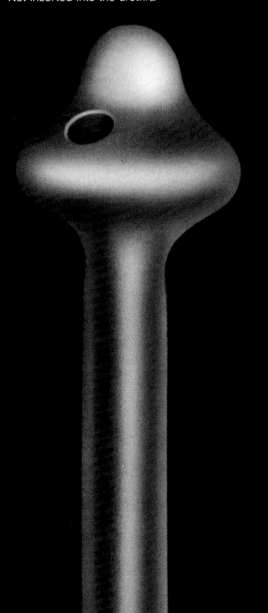

Malecot (bat-wing)
A single-lumen straight catheter with a winged tip (similar to the mushroom-shaped tip except with wedges taken out of it).

Use
• To provide for bladder drainage as a suprapubic tube
• To provide for kidney drainage as a flank tube

Special considerations
• Must be inserted with the aid of a stylet, which temporarily straightens out the tip.
• Usually sutured in place
• Not inserted into the urethra

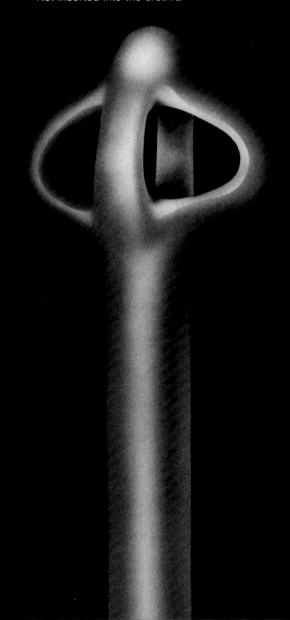

Surgical care

Caring for a postop urology patient

No matter what type of urinary tract surgery your patient had, you should follow these general postop procedures:
• Check any indwelling catheters for patency immediately after the patient returns to your care. Make sure all catheter and tubing connections are secure and draining. For the first 24 hours following surgery, check the patient's urine flow hourly. This will ensure against leaving the drainage tube blocked for a dangerous period of time. If the catheter seems obstructed, notify the doctor.

If your hospital policy allows you to irrigate an indwelling catheter and the doctor expressly orders you to do so, would you know how? Follow these instructions. Irrigate a suprapubic catheter as you would an indwelling urethral catheter (see page 46). Irrigate a flank catheter this way: First, try rolling the catheter between your fingers to free the obstruction. If this doesn't work, get a 5 cc sy-

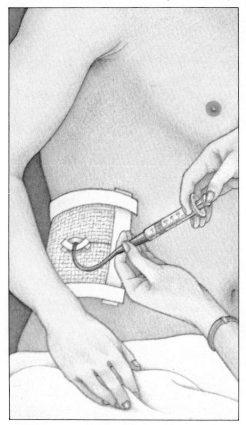

ringe filled with sterile normal saline solution. Insert the syringe into the catheter and slowly instill about 2 ml saline solution, or more if ordered. Then, slowly aspirate the solution.

Important: Use extreme caution during this procedure to avoid causing kidney damage. If this doesn't unclog the tube, alert the doctor.
• Record the patient's fluid intake and output for at least 3 days postop. The doctor may

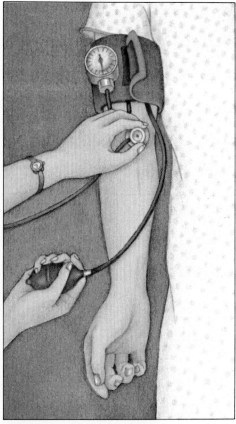

want him to drink as much as 3,000 ml fluid daily. Administer it carefully, watching your patient for signs of abdominal distention. If distention occurs, the doctor will discontinue the patient's oral intake and may order the insertion of a nasogastric tube.

Usually, the patient will begin a regular diet 4 days postop.
• Monitor your patient's fluid and electrolyte levels. Consult the chart on page 80 to learn the signs of imbalance. If you suspect a fluid or electrolyte imbalance, notify the doctor. He'll probably order an I.V. solution with the proper ionic proportions to restore balance.
• Every 2 hours, monitor your patient's temperature, blood pressure, pulse, and respirations. He may develop a mild fever, but don't let this alarm you. It may be the usual response to surgery or inadequate hydration. But, if your patient's temperature reaches 101° F. (38.3° C.) and is accompanied by chills, call the doctor. This may indicate infection and should be treated immediately.
• Watch for signs of hemorrhage. They include tachycardia, hypotension, apprehension, and pallid, cold, clammy skin. To evaluate hypotension, use the patient's preop blood pressure as a reference point. But, remember, the preop blood pressure may differ from what's considered normal. Also, if his urine

is bright red, his blood pressure drops, his pulse becomes rapid and thready, or his skin becomes clammy or pale, suspect internal hemorrhage. In such a case, notify the doctor immediately. If the bleeding's at the suture site, immediately apply a pressure dressing to the incision.
• Check the patient's draining urine for color, clarity, odor, and amount. Record your observations and report any abnormalities to the doctor. If you don't observe any abnormalities the first 24 hours postop, check the patient's urine at least once every 8 hours thereafter.

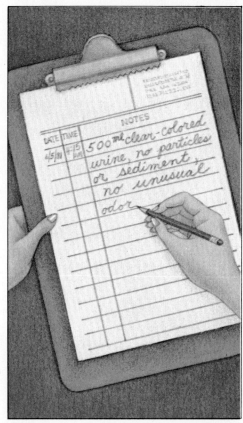

• Change the dressing around the catheter at least once a day or whenever it becomes wet or soiled. Do this following the instructions on pages 84 and 85. Observe strict aseptic technique. If irrigation's also necessary, do it before you change the dressing.
• Care for a Penrose drain as you would a urine drainage tube. If drainage from the incision becomes copious, attach an ostomy bag to the drain site. Care for the bag as you would for a normal ostomy bag.
• Check the incision for signs of infection (redness, turgor, warmth, purulent drainage). If dehiscence or bowel evisceration occurs, notify the doctor. For more details on these complications, see page 101. Administer antibiotics, as ordered.

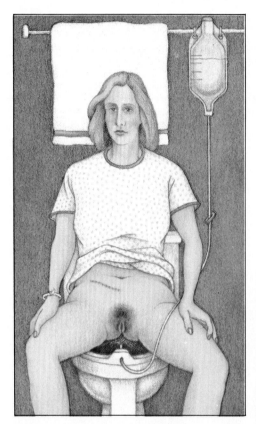

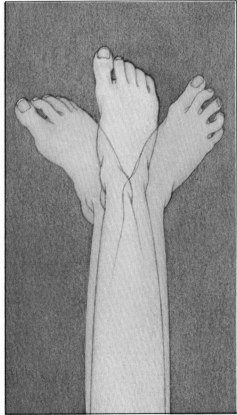

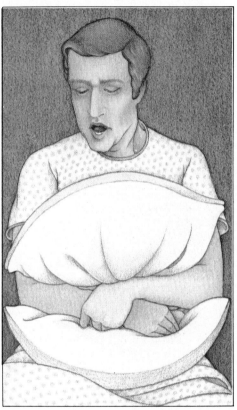

• Give mild cathartics or stool softeners, as ordered, to minimize bowel straining. You probably won't give an enema because it will irritate the colon.

• Give pain medications for 48 hours postop, as ordered. For the patient with severe back pain from flank surgery, the doctor will probably order a muscle relaxant. For full effectiveness, give the medication before the pain becomes severe.

• If your patient's had lower urinary tract surgery, suspect bladder spasms if he complains of intermittent or constant pain (but his urine flow remains normal). Spasms are not dangerous and should subside within a day or two. In the meantime, ease your patient's discomfort with an antispasmodic medication or a sitz bath.

• Don't allow the patient to sit in a chair for extended periods of time. This causes greater stasis of venous blood flow to his legs and pelvis than bed rest does. To prevent thrombus formation, the doctor will probably order these exercises for your patient: rotating his ankle, flexing his knee, and pressing the back of his knee to the mattress. Follow the schedule that the doctor orders. Barring complications, he'll usually allow the patient to ambulate 24 hours following surgery.

• Encourage the patient who's had flank sur-

gery to perform the deep breathing, coughing, and turning exercises you taught him preop. The doctor may have applied an abdominal binder following surgery to help splint the incision when the patient coughs. If the patient doesn't have an abdominal binder, show him how to splint his chest with a pillow. The doctor may also order incentive spirometry therapy to help your patient breathe deeply.

• Discontinue the suprapubic catheter following doctor's orders. This involves clamping the catheter until the patient complains of bladder discomfort. At this point, the catheter's unclamped, allowing the bladder to drain. Then, it's clamped again. The procedure's repeated until the patient urinates and leaves minimal (less than 20 ml) residual urine in his bladder. Then the doctor will order catheter removal.

• Depending on your patient's surgery, you may have to give him additional postop care. Turn the page to learn about some extra responsibilities that you'll have in caring for such a patient. Then, to learn about specific care techniques for the patient who has undergone urinary diversion, refer to the section on ostomy care. Finally, turn to the last section of this book to find detailed information on caring for the dialysis patient and the renal transplant patient.

Surgical care

Caring for the postop urology patient: Special considerations

As we've shown on the preceding two pages, your responsibilities in postop urologic care are broad and detailed. But, depending on the specific surgery your patient's had, you may have additional responsibilities. Consider these points:
• If your female patient's had urethral surgery, don't dress her perineal incision with gauze pads or allow her to wear panties. Either may irritate the incision. If the doctor orders, remove any urethral catheter 24 hours postop. Upon removal, observe the meatus for bleeding and notify the doctor if you see any.
• If your patient's had a transurethral resection (TUR), save his first independently urinated specimen for examination, if the doctor orders.
• If your patient's had a radical perineal prostatectomy, show him how to clean his perineum with antibacterial solution after each bowel movement; also, how to change his dressing. Tell him how to do exercises to strengthen his perineum. Provide him with counseling if the surgery renders him temporarily or permanently incontinent. Assure him that fecal incontinence is usually temporary.
• If your patient's had bladder surgery, you may be instructed to insert a nasogastric tube into your patient's stomach to periodically suction him. To learn how, see the NURSING PHOTO-BOOK PERFORMING GI PROCEDURES.
• If your patient's had kidney surgery, you may be instructed to administer neostigmine methylsulfate (Prostigmin*) and to insert a rectal tube to relieve abdominal distention. For details on how to insert a rectal tube, see the NURSING PHOTOBOOK PERFORMING GI PROCEDURES. Remember, never leave a rectal tube in place for more than 20 minutes.

Maintaining your patient's fluid and electrolyte balance

Since you're responsible for notifying the doctor if the patient has a fluid or electrolyte imbalance, you must know what to look for. This list details the various imbalances you're likely to find and how to distinguish between them.

Dehydration	Loose, flushed, dry skin, shriveled and dry-looking tongue, sunken eyes, low urine output, high specific gravity, excessive thirst
Overhydration	Restlessness, dependent edema, pulmonary rales, dyspnea, indicating congestive heart failure or pulmonary edema
Hyponatremia	Nausea, headaches, muscular weakness, hyperreflexia, abdominal cramps, nausea, vomiting, diarrhea
Hypernatremia	Restlessness, tachycardia, edema, hyperreflexia
Hypokalemia	Weakness, apprehension, paralysis, nausea, vomiting, abdominal distention, cardiac arrhythmias, convulsions, coma
Hyperkalemia	Nausea, diarrhea, abdominal cramps, muscular weakness, irregular pulse
Hypocalcemia	Renal failure, paresthesia, muscle irritability, tetany, convulsions, hyperreflexia, numbness and tingling of nose, ears, fingertips, and toes
Hypercalcemia	Excessive thirst, lethargy, mental confusion, nausea, vomiting, constipation
Acidosis	Deep breathing, fruity odor to breath, disorientation, headache, drowsiness, stupor, coma
Alkalosis	Hyperventilation, light-headedness, tetany, syncope

*Available in both the United States and in Canada

Performing continuous bladder irrigation

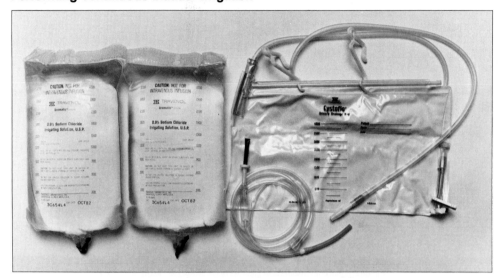

1 *Mr. Alfred Norwood has just returned from a transurethral resection with an indwelling (Foley) catheter in his urethra. If the doctor ordered intermittent bladder irrigation, you'd turn to page 46 to find out how it's done. But instead, he wants you to begin continuous irrigation of Mr. Norwood's bladder to ensure against blood clotting and to promote healing. Do you know how continuous irrigation's done?*

Begin by gathering this equipment: 4,000 ml drainage bag, continuous bladder irrigation tubing, and two 3,000 ml bags normal saline solution for irrigation (one for immediate use and one for later use). You'll also need an I.V. pole, sterile gloves, and an emesis basin.

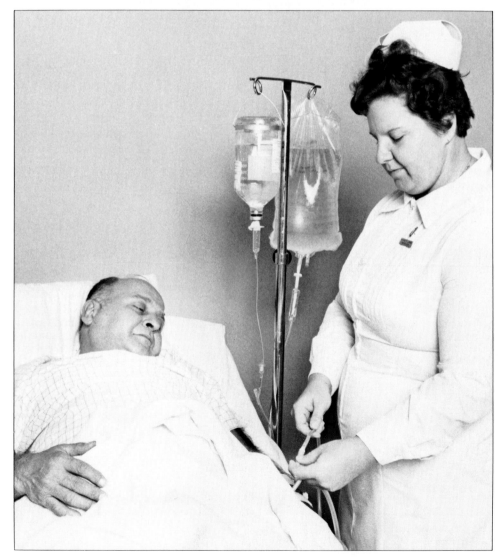

2 Provide privacy for this procedure. Explain to Mr. Norwood why irrigating his bladder's important and how it's done. Then, wash your hands. Since Mr. Norwood has an I.V. line in place, the I.V. pole's already at his bedside. Hang the saline solution on the pole.

Surgical care

Performing continuous bladder irrigation continued

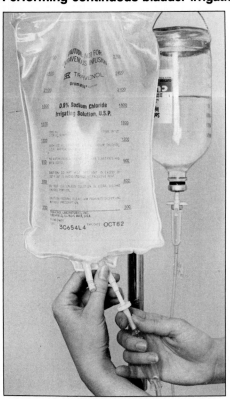

3 Close the clamp on the irrigation tubing. Spike the irrigation bag with the irrigation tubing.

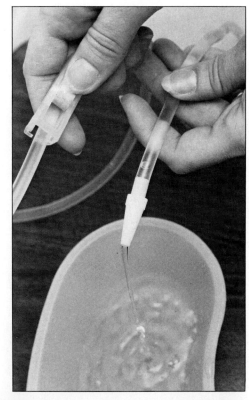

4 Position the end of the irrigation tubing over the emesis basin. Open the clamp to allow the irrigation solution to run through the tubing and remove all air. Then, reclamp the tubing.

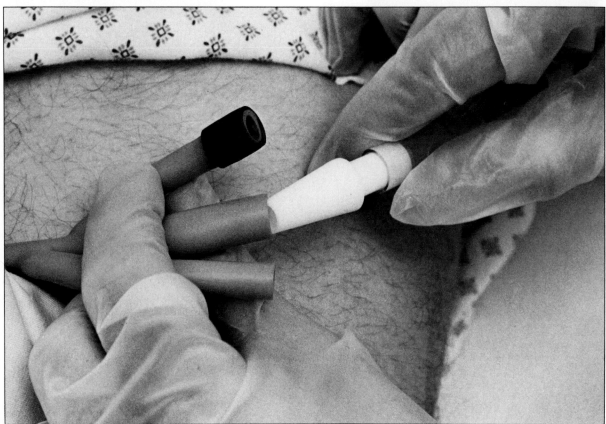

5 Put on sterile gloves. Disconnect the Foley drainage tubing from the large lumen of the three-way Foley catheter and cap the tubing. Unplug the small lumen of the three-way Foley catheter. Then, take the tubing of the 4,000 ml drainage bag and connect it to the large lumen of the Foley catheter, as shown here. Use the aseptic procedure described on pages 43 and 44.

6 Next, connect the irrigation tubing to the small lumen of the Foley catheter, as the nurse is doing here.

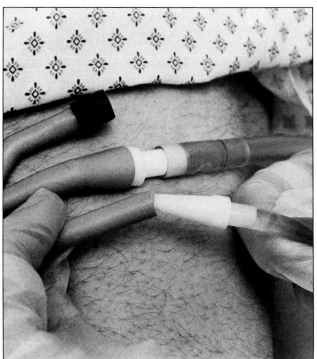

7 Open the clamp on the irrigation tubing and adjust the flow rate. This will let the irrigation solution flow into the bladder then out to the drainage bag.

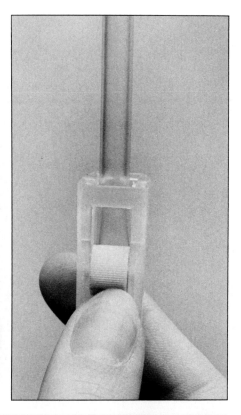

8 When the irrigation solution bag is almost empty, replace it, interrupting bladder irrigation only long enough to repeat the hanging, priming, and connecting procedure just detailed. Since you can reuse the irrigation tubing, you don't need to adjust the flow rate.

When the drainage bag becomes full, empty it as you would a conventional Foley drainage bag, as shown on page 41.

When the doctor orders the end to the continuous bladder irrigation procedure, remove the drainage bag and replace it with a conventional Foley drainage bag. Cap or plug the small lumen of the Foley catheter.

Throughout the irrigation procedure, record the patient's intake and output. Also record the color and amount of the urine, presence of blood clots, how the patient tolerated the procedure, and the date and time irrigation began and ended.

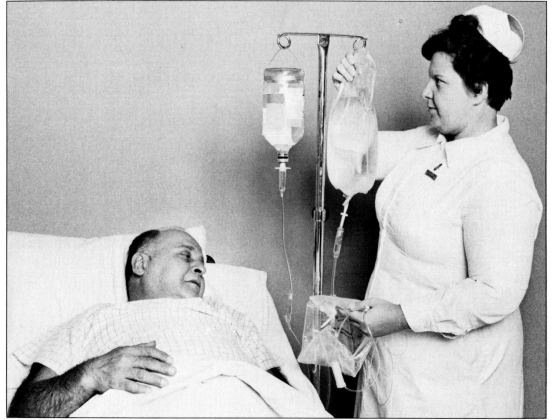

Surgical care

Changing a drainage-tube dressing

1 *Whenever the dressing around your patient's suprapubic tube becomes wet or soiled, remove and replace it. The procedure is simple, but must be done with care. Here's how:*
First, assemble the equipment shown here. Make sure the tape you use is nonallergenic. Also, bring a paper bag with you to put the old dressing in.

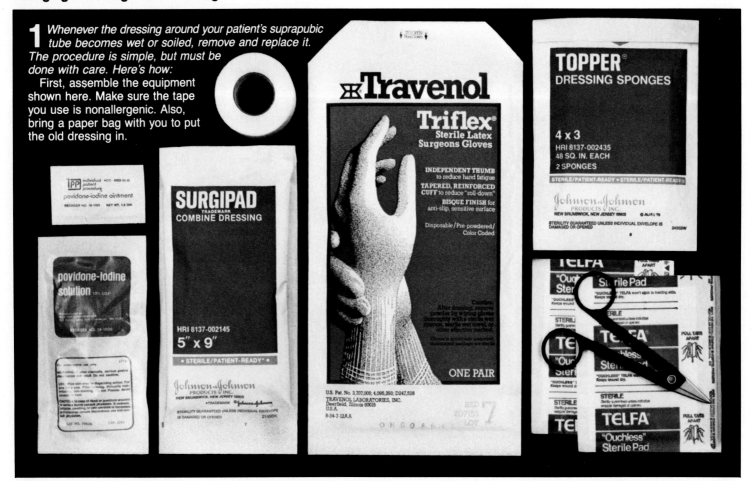

2 Wash your hands. Then, explain the procedure to the patient.
Gently remove the old dressing. Try not to jar the catheter or you might cause the patient to have a bladder spasm. If you have difficulty removing the dressing, try saturating it with sterile saline solution (see inset photo). Let it soak for 5 minutes. Then, remove the dressing and thoroughly dry the site. Place the old dressing in the paper bag. Remove the bag when you leave.

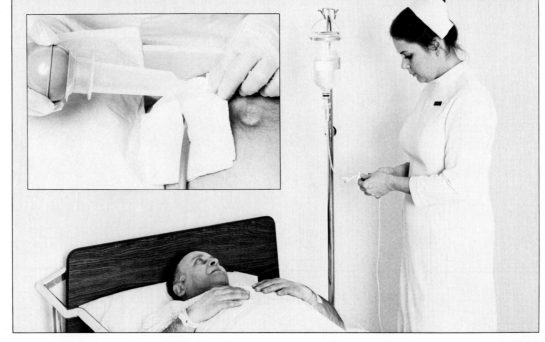

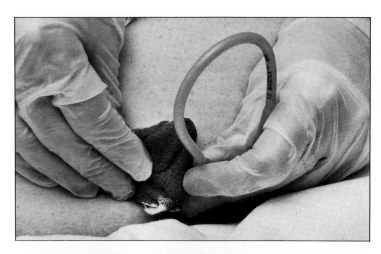

3 Examine the patient's incision. If it's red, hard, malodorous, or has purulent drainage, notify the doctor. Then, put on sterile gloves and clean the incision with povidone-iodine solution. Use a circular motion and move outward from the catheter. This way you avoid sweeping contaminants into the incision. Let the solution dry before proceeding. Then, apply a small amount of Betadine ointment around the insertion site.

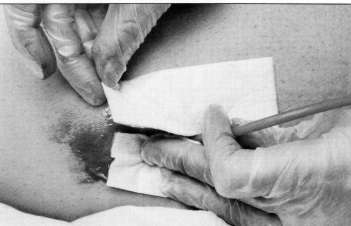

4 Place two precut Telfa®-coated pads around the catheter and over the incision. If the pads you're using aren't precut, cut them yourself. Do this by placing one on top of the other. Using sterile scissors, start at the midpoint of one side and cut 2″ into the pads.

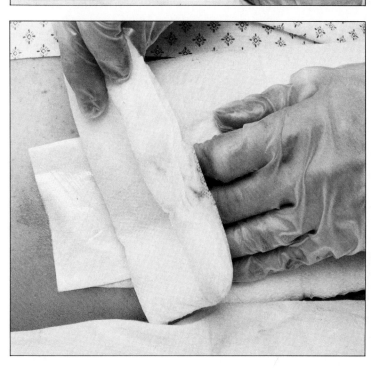

5 Then, place a sterile Surgipad™ over the Telfa-coated pads and the catheter. Tape the Surgipad in place with nonallergenic tape. Finally, record your actions on the patient's chart and in your nurses' notes.

Learning about stress incontinence

What's stress incontinence? It's a condition affecting the endopelvic fascial muscles of older women. These muscles, which support the bladder, weaken with age and the stress of childbirth to such an extent that when the patient exerts or strains herself, incontinence occurs.

This condition, in its most serious form, involves total bladder extrusion. In such a case, the doctor will probably instruct you to apply, preop, continuous saline soaks to the protruding bladder, to treat or prevent ulceration.

To repair weakened endopelvic fascial muscles, the doctor will place the patient in the Trendelenberg or the lithotomy position and make an incision in the wall of the vagina to expose the muscles. He'll strengthen these muscles by tightening them with sutures. Then, he'll suture the vaginal wall and leave a vaginal pack and urethral catheter in place. He'll probably order the vaginal pack removed in 24 hours and the catheter removed in 7 days.

How do you care postoperatively for this patient? You'll provide general urinary tract postop care, paying particular attention to keeping the urethral catheter patent. If clotting occurs, the patient's urine will back up and strain the sutured muscles. During immediate postop, teach the patient muscle exercises, as you would for a postop transurethral resection (TUR) patient, to strengthen her perineal muscles. Finally, check the vaginal pack frequently to make sure it doesn't work its way up or out the vaginal canal.

Surgical care

Learning about penile implants

Patient care

Roger Ellison, a 54-year-old high-school teacher, has been hospitalized for penile implant surgery. He's getting the implant to make his penis erect, so he can have sexual intercourse. What caused his impotence? Probably one of these things: diabetes, an emotional or psychologic problem, or spinal cord damage from pelvic injury or surgery. Whatever the reason, Mr. Ellison's age is typical for this surgery; most patients are between ages 40 and 69.

Mr. Ellison and his doctor have discussed the two basic types of penile implants available: silicone rods and inflatable silicone-rubber cylinders. You can learn the pros and cons of each by reading the information to the right.

Make sure Mr. Ellison knows that both implant methods carry infection risks and cause discomfort. How long that discomfort lasts depends primarily on the degree of tissue trauma caused by the surgery. He should also know that periodically he may need additional surgery—particularly if he's getting an inflatable implant—to remove or replace defective parts.

During the patient's recovery (if your hospital directs), tell him to wear loose-fitting underwear and clothing so he doesn't put prolonged pressure on the end of his penis.

Before the patient goes home, he should be given these instructions:
• Tell him to call his doctor if he develops a temperature of 101° F. (38.3° C.) or more; if the pain he feels gets worse; or if his penis becomes sore or drains pus.
• Tell him to avoid sexual activity for at least 6 weeks after the surgery, to allow the incision to heal.
• Have him ask the doctor when he'll be able to return to work.

Silicone rod implants

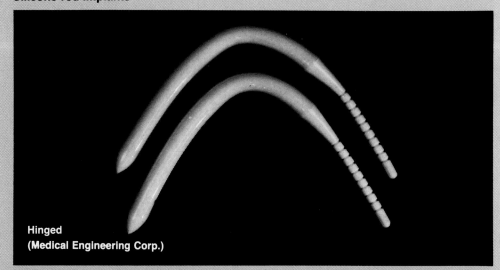

Hinged
(Medical Engineering Corp.)

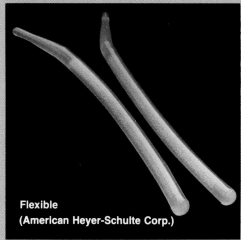

Flexible
(American Heyer-Schulte Corp.)

Wire
(Dacomed Corp.)

Description

Two silicone-rubber rods implanted within the corpora cavernosa of the penis. These rods come in three basic varieties: hinged, flexible, and wire. The hinged type has a hinge as part of its construction. The flexible type is a foam-filled silicone rod. The wire type has silver wire strands twisted together to form a silver core within the rod.

Advantages
• Minor surgery
• Simple device
• Inexpensive device

Disadvantages
• Permanent erection, with flexible and hinged types, may cause cosmetic problems.
• Silicone rod may fracture, requiring replacement.
• Permanent erection, with flexible and hinged types, may weaken surrounding tissue, because undergarments press penis against body.

Nursing considerations
• Administer broad-spectrum antibiotics, to prevent infection, as ordered.
• Relieve postop urinary retention with intermittent catheterization using a small-lumen Robinson catheter.
• Watch for these complications: incision infection, priapism, or implant extrusion.

Inflatable implant

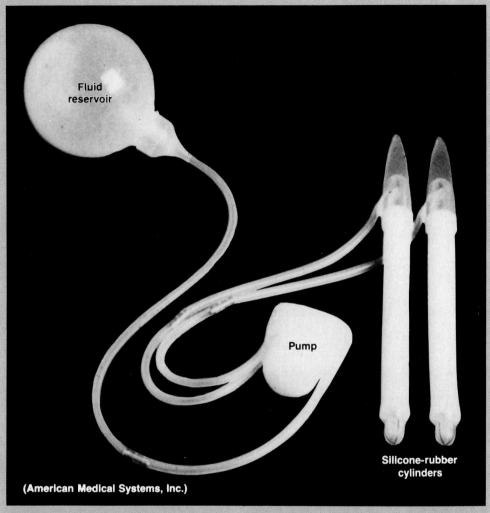

Fluid reservoir

Pump

Silicone-rubber cylinders

(American Medical Systems, Inc.)

Description

Two silicone-rubber cylinders placed on either side of the penile shaft. The patient manually inflates these cylinders with fluid using a pump and valve device implanted in the scrotum. The fluid's contained in a round reservoir that's implanted near the bladder.

Advantages

• Voluntary erection

Disadvantages

• Major surgery
• Mechanical complications may require additional surgery for repairs.
• Inconvenient manual inflation
• Unequal filling of rods possible
• Asymmetrical filling of rods possible
• Expensive device

Nursing considerations

• Instruct the patient in pump bulb manipulation as early as 6 days postop.
• Administer broad-spectrum antibiotics, as ordered, to prevent infection.
• Relieve postop urinary retention with intermittent catheterization using a small-lumen Robinson catheter.
• Watch for these complications: incision infection and priapism.

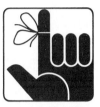

PATIENT TEACHING

Teaching a patient to care for himself

While your patient's hospitalized, you'll give him the best care you can. But what happens when he goes home and you're not there to care for him? You must teach him how to care for himself and make him understand the importance of maintaining that self-care.

If he's going home with an indwelling (Foley) catheter in place, refer to pages 51 to 53 for information you can teach and send home with him. If your patient has an ostomy, turn to the ostomy section of this book. There you'll find how you can help him make a successful adjustment to his changed body image. If your patient's had kidney transplant surgery, reading the final section of this book will give you insight into his condition and show you how to teach him self-care.

The home care aids on the following pages (adapted from those used by the James A. Haley Veterans Administration Hospital in Tampa, Florida) focus on the do's and don'ts of exercise and diet for the patient who's had kidney, bladder, prostate, or scrotal surgery.

Patient teaching

Home care

After scrotal surgery: How to care for yourself

Dear Patient:

As you know, you've just had surgery on your scrotum. By observing a few important precautions, you can help speed your recovery. Read the list that follows. If you have any questions, talk to your nurse. Then, when you go home, make a special effort to follow the guidelines listed here:

• Restrict your activities. For example, take only short walks, and climb no more than 2 flights of stairs at a time. Don't lift or carry heavy objects for at least 4 weeks.

• If you develop any increased soreness, redness, or swelling around the site, or if the incision drainage increases, call your doctor. Wear a scrotal support or briefs for at least 3 weeks to help prevent or minimize swelling.

• Do not engage in any sexual activity for at least 6 weeks after the operation.

• If your temperature is 101° F. (38.3° C.) or more, call your doctor.

• If your scrotum becomes bruised, don't become alarmed. This is normal and will gradually disappear. Any discomfort can be lessened by taking a sitz bath. You can obtain a prepackaged sitz bath kit or you can take a sitz bath at home using only your bathtub. Here's how:

Fill the tub with a few inches of warm water. Then, sit in the tub and let the water bathe your scrotum for at least 20 minutes. Add extra water to keep it warm.

• If your surgery was for sterilization, you will return to the hospital for two consecutive laboratory tests, taken 1 month apart. These tests will confirm sterility by determining the sperm content of your ejaculate.

• At your next doctor's appointment, ask your doctor when you can return to work. This will vary depending on your health, your job, and the surgery you've had.

Home care

After prostate surgery: How to care for yourself

Dear Patient:

You've just had surgery on your prostate gland. To speed your recovery, observe these precautions:

• Restrict your activities. For example, take only short walks and climb no more than 2 flights of stairs at a time. Ride in a car as little as possible during the first 3 weeks, because vehicle motion may strain your bladder. Don't lift heavy objects for at least 3 weeks.

• Drink 12 to 14 8-oz. glasses of liquid each day, unless the doctor orders otherwise.

• Don't become alarmed if you see some blood in your urine during the first 2 weeks after surgery. But, if you see blood, drink some fluid and lie down. The next time you urinate, the bleeding should decrease. If it doesn't, call your doctor. If your urine stream diminishes or if you can't urinate at all, notify your doctor. Don't worry if you lose some control over urination, if you feel pain, or if you have a frequent need to urinate. These symptoms will

disappear with time.

• To strengthen your perineal muscles, perform this exercise: Press your buttocks together. Hold this position a few seconds, then relax. Repeat 10 times in succession, _____times a day.

• Don't strain to have a bowel movement. If you're constipated, take a laxative. Don't give yourself an enema or place anything—for example, a suppository—into your rectum for 4 weeks after surgery.

• Avoid sexual activity for 4 weeks after surgery because it can cause bleeding. When you do engage in sex, most of your sperm will go into your bladder instead of out your penis. This will cause your urine to be cloudy and will decrease, though not end, your fertility. You will still experience orgasm.

• At your next doctor's appointment, ask when you can return to work. This will vary depending on your health, your job, and the type of surgery you've had.

Home care

After bladder surgery: How to care for yourself

Dear Patient:

As you know, you've just had surgery on your bladder. To speed your recovery, observe these precautions:

• Empty your bladder at least once every 2 hours. Never let your bladder become full.

• Take frequent short walks. This will improve your urine flow. But don't overtire yourself.

• Drink 12 to 14 8-oz. glasses of water each day, unless your doctor orders otherwise. Increase the amount you drink at night to prevent your urine from becoming too concentrated.

• When you urinate, you may feel some burning or pain, but this should disappear with time. You may also see some blood in your urine. If you do see blood, drink some fluid and lie down for a while. The next time you urinate, the bleeding should be decreased. If it hasn't, or if it increases, call your doctor. If your urine stream diminishes or stops completely (and you still feel the urge to urinate), call your doctor.

• Never strain to have a bowel movement. Take a mild laxative if you get constipated. Don't give yourself an enema or put anything in your rectum (for example, a suppository) for 4 weeks.

• Avoid riding in a car or other moving vehicle for 3 weeks. Vehicle motion can strain your bladder.

• Do not lift or carry heavy objects or engage in strenuous physical activity for at least 4 weeks or you'll cause bleeding.

• Call your doctor if your temperature is 101° F. (38.3° C.) or more, or if you see pus in your urine.

• Don't salt your food because salt promotes water retention, which affects kidney function. Reduce the amount of calcium- and phosphorus-rich foods you eat, such as dairy products, shellfish, and dark green vegetables. This will reduce your chance of developing bladder stones.

• At your next doctor's appointment, ask when you can return to work. This will vary, depending on your health, your job, and the surgery you've had.

Home care

After kidney surgery: How to care for yourself

Dear Patient:

As you recover from kidney surgery, you can expect to feel discomfort in your side for 4 to 6 weeks, but this discomfort will gradually disappear. You may find that the pain moves from your side to your front. This is normal. But, if it increases, call your doctor. You may also have swelling or numbness near or below the incision. This will go away during your convalescence. Follow these precautions to speed your recovery:

• Drink 12 to 14 8-oz. glasses of fluid each day, unless the doctor orders otherwise. Drink even more during summer months if you sweat a lot. Increase the amount you drink at night to prevent your urine from becoming too concentrated. If your kidney surgery was done for a reason other than removing stones, drink your usual amount of water.

• Take frequent short walks. This will improve your urine flow. But discontinue these walks if they begin overtiring you.

• Don't salt your food because salt promotes water retention, which affects kidney function. To reduce your chance of developing kidney stones, reduce the amount of calcium- and phosphorus-rich foods you eat, such as dairy products, shellfish, and dark green vegetables. Ask for the hospital dietitian if you have any questions about diet.

• Do not lift or carry any heavy objects for at least 4 weeks.

• Call your doctor if you notice an increase in drainage from the incision. When you no longer have any drainage, you can stop wearing a dressing.

• Call your doctor if your temperature is 101° F. (38.3° C.) or more. In such a case, drink extra fluid and get plenty of rest.

• At your next doctor's appointment, ask when you can return to work. Recovery time varies depending on your health, your job, and the type of surgery you've had.

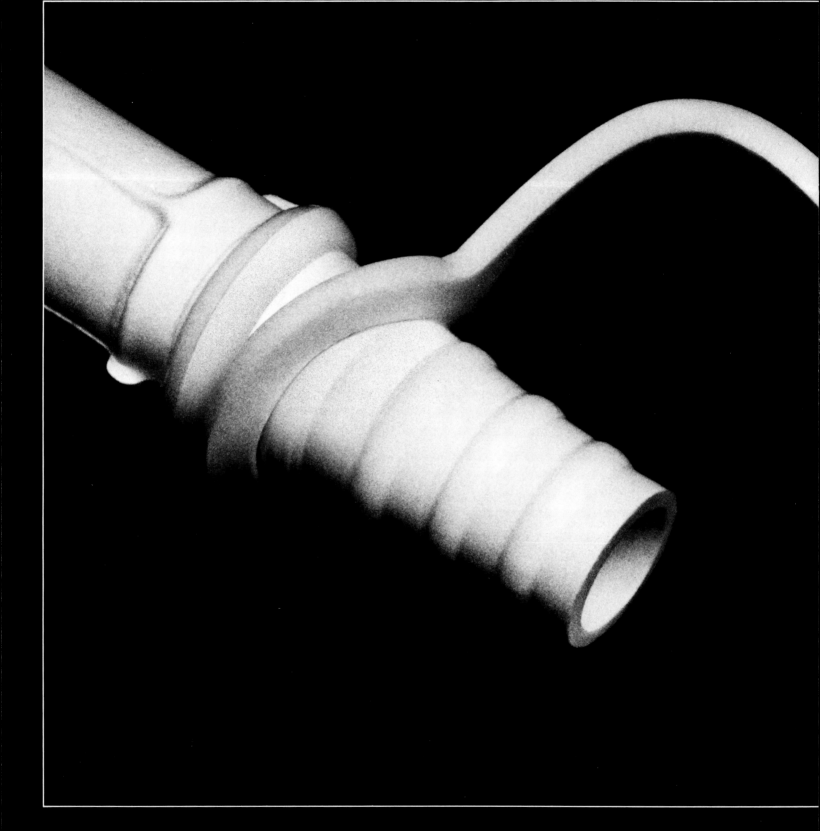

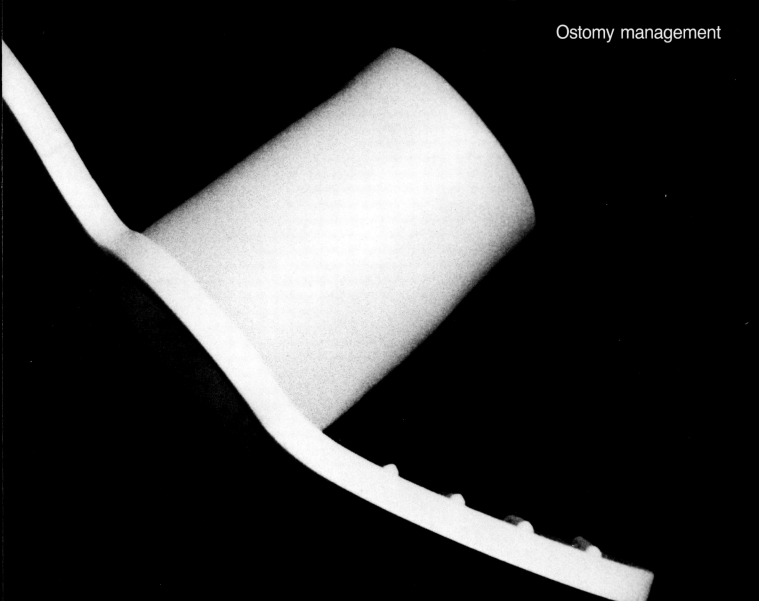

Caring for the Ostomy Patient

Ostomy management

Ostomy management

When the doctor performs urinary diversion surgery, he'll usually create a stoma. What are your responsibilities in caring for the patient with an ostomy? Consider these:
- preparing the patient for surgery
- applying a reusable or disposable ostomy pouch
- caring for the stoma and peristomal area
- dealing with common ostomy complications
- rehabilitating your patient
- teaching the patient home care
- teaching the continent-vesicostomy patient self-catheterization technique.

In the pages that follow, we'll detail these responsibilities, and provide you with tips to make the tasks easier.

When urinary diversion surgery's indicated

As you know, urinary ostomy surgery is done to divert urine from a damaged or diseased bladder and to drain it, instead, from a stoma, which the doctor forms in the abdominal wall. The doctor may perform urinary diversion surgery if your patient's:
- a child with a congenital urinary tract defect.
- a child with a urinary tract infection so severe that permanent kidney damage could result if the operation isn't performed.
- an adult with a severely diseased urinary tract.
- an adult with an injured urinary tract.
- an injured adult, for example, a paraplegic, whose care would be made easier by having an ostomy.

Learning about different urinary diversion surgeries

ILEAL CONDUIT (ileal loop)

Description

The doctor excises a small portion of the ileum, anastomosing the remaining intestine to restore intestinal integrity. He dissects the ureters from the bladder and anastomoses them to the ileal segment. He closes one end of the ileal segment with sutures, and brings the other end through the abdominal wall, forming a stoma.

Advantages

- Minimal urine reflux because the ileal segment stays virtually emptied
- Minimal absorption of urinary electrolytes
- Easy to care for and fit with faceplate

Disadvantages

- Can't be used if patient's blood urea nitrogen (BUN) level is 40% above normal.
- Moderate chance of postop complications

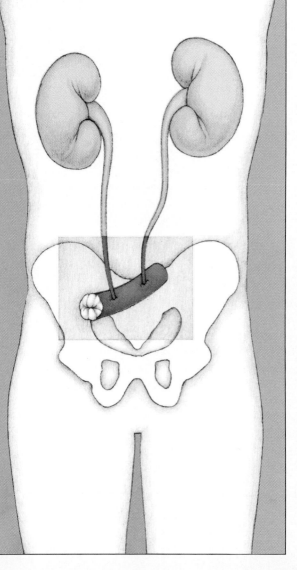

CONTINENT VESICOSTOMY

Description

- The doctor forms a tube from part of the bladder wall. He brings one end of the tube to the skin to form a stoma. Then, he sutures the patient's urethra closed.

Advantages

- Good urinary control
- No need for external urine collection since stoma remains closed from bladder pressure

Disadvantages

- Requires bladder that's free of disease.

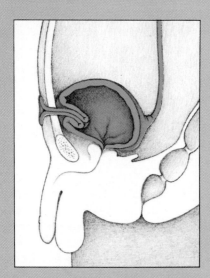

Preparing your patient for ostomy surgery

Some hospitals delegate preoperative ostomy teaching to an enterostomal therapist, but your hospital may make you responsible for the preparation procedure. What should you do? We'll tell you.

Even if the doctor has explained to your patient what the diagnosis means and what surgery's involved, you may discover the patient still doesn't understand what's going to happen to him. Review the procedure with him using anatomical illustrations of the urinary tract. How much detail should you provide? To answer this, judge your patient's needs. One patient may want extensive information on his condition. In such a case, provide what you can and supplement it with booklets from the United Ostomy Association. Another patient may not want much information. Tell him only the essentials; for example, that his stoma will drain urine and that he'll have to wear a pouch. Save the rest for postoperative teaching. At that time, you may also want to suggest special counseling—for example, sexual—for the patient having difficulty adjusting to his condition.

In any event, prepare your patient for the stoma's appearance. He should know it will be red and moist, and may bleed a bit postoperatively. For the patient who wishes to know more about stoma care or seems upset about having a stoma, show him a pouch. Describe how easily the pouch fits over the stoma and how trouble-free it is to manage. You may find that you can further ease your patient's apprehensions by reassuring him that later he'll get complete training on how to care for his stoma.

As you teach, listen to your patient so you can discover some of his fears. Correct any misconceptions he has; for example, tell the patient with a previously satisfying sex life that he'll probably be able to resume it following surgery. As another example, tell the female ostomate she'll still be able to bear children. Never lie to your patient, but be as positive as possible about his future lifestyle. You may find the most effective way to relieve his fears is by inviting a well-adjusted ostomate of the same sex and age to visit him. No one is better prepared to relate to your patient's problems. If the doctor says it's okay, contact the United Ostomy Association for help in selecting an appropriate ostomy visitor.

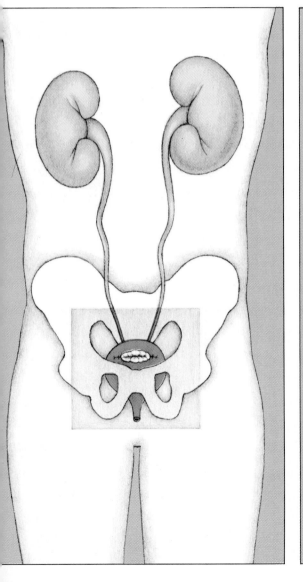

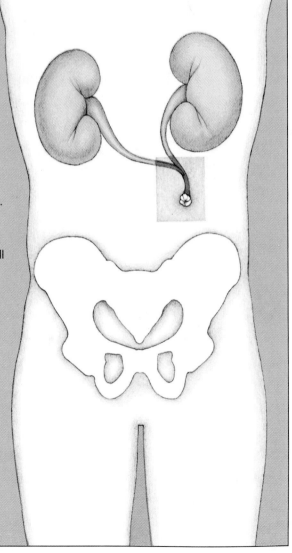

CUTANEOUS URETEROSTOMY

Description
The doctor dissects one or both ureters from the bladder and brings them to the skin, forming one or two stomas.

Advantages
• Less complicated, less time consuming, and less stressful to patient than ileal conduit
• Works successfully with thick-walled, chronically dilated ureters.

Disadvantages
• Difficult to care for and fit with faceplate, because stoma is small and almost flush with skin
• High chance of ureter stricture

Ostomy management

Selecting a stoma site

How will the doctor or enterostomal therapist (ET) decide where to locate your patient's stoma? His primary consideration, of course, will be the condition of the patient's urinary tract (which may not be known until surgery). However, he'll probably also consider the following: type of surgery, previous incisions, scars, skin folds, bony prominences, and belt line. He'll also observe the patient lying, sitting, and standing. If the stoma location isn't dictated by any of the above considerations, the doctor or ET will work with the patient to select the site, which is desirable because the patient's given some control over his future appearance.

Usually, the doctor will construct the stoma at the center of one of two triangles formed by these imaginary lines:
• from the umbilicus to the symphysis pubis, to the iliac crest and back to the umbilicus. This site, the one most commonly selected, places the stoma below the patient's waistline.
• from the umbilicus to the iliac crest, to the xyphoid process and back to the umbilicus. This site places the stoma above the waistline.

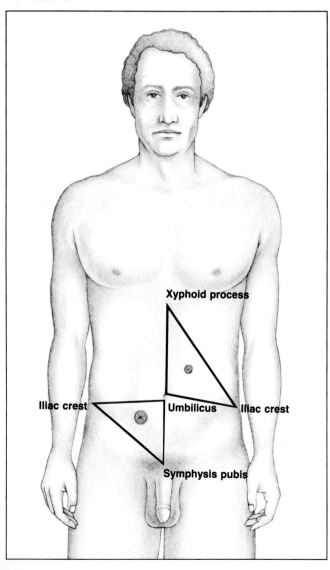

Xyphoid process

Iliac crest   Umbilicus   Iliac crest

Symphysis pubis

Selecting a stoma pouch

You or the enterostomal therapist will select a pouch that suits your patient's needs. In doing so, consider such things as the type of ostomy, the shape and location of the stoma, the patient's physical and mental competence, his financial situation, his future physical activities, his skin allergies and sensitivities, and the size and contour of his body. This chart weighs the advantages and disadvantages of the various pouches available.

The pediatric patient will be outfitted with a pouch that's designed to fit his size and body shape. With an infant, you may use a diaper instead of a pouch.

What's the ultimate test of a pouch's suitability? Whether or not it works. In most cases, a pouch will adhere to the patient's skin for at least 2 days. However, it may require a week of frequent applications to accomplish this. At that point, if no peristomal skin excoriation is present, the patient's probably found the pouch that's right for him.

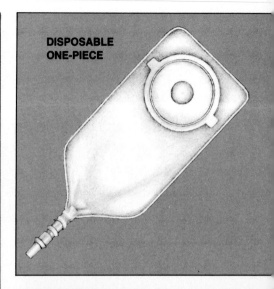

DISPOSABLE ONE-PIECE

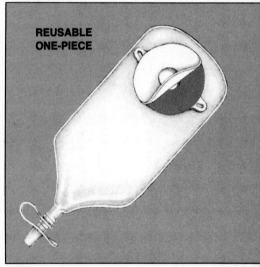

REUSABLE ONE-PIECE

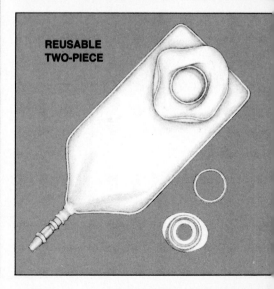

REUSABLE TWO-PIECE

Description

Vinyl pouch, attached to adhesive-backed faceplate. May or may not be precut. Used with skin barrier.

Advantages
- Easy to apply
- Easy to maintain

Disadvantages
- Most expensive method

Description

Vinyl pouch attached to opaque faceplate with insert adaptable to stoma size. Used with skin barrier. May or may not have belt attachment.

Advantages
- Easy to use for those with poor vision or diminished manual dexterity
- Durable
- Less expensive than disposable

Disadvantages
- More expensive than reusable two-piece pouch
- Bulkiest
- Most demanding to maintain

Description

Vinyl pouch, separate opaque faceplate with adaptable insert to fit stoma. Used with skin barrier. May or may not have belt attachment.

Advantages
- Can see stoma and change pouch without removing faceplate.
- Lighter, less bulky, and less expensive than one-piece reusable pouch

Disadvantages
- Most difficult to apply
- More demanding to maintain than disposable one-piece pouch

Caring for the stoma and peristomal area

Basically, your ostomy care responsibilities are twofold; stoma and peristomal care. Stomas come in a variety of shapes and sizes. Some protrude from the skin in budlike fashion. Others remain flush with the skin. You'll find that fitting a faceplate to a budlike stoma is easiest. However, you can make a flush stoma protrude a little by using a convex faceplate. Then it will be almost as easy to fit as a budlike stoma.

Your patient's stoma should stay bright red. If it becomes deep red or bluish, suspect a problem in the blood supply and notify the doctor. Expect the stoma to bleed a little when touched, particularly just after surgery. But since the stoma has no nerve endings, this temporary condition will not cause your patient discomfort.

Depending on your hospital's policy, and doctor's orders, you may have to dilate your patient's stoma periodically. To do this, put a sterile glove on your hand or put a finger cot on your little finger. Lubricate your little finger and insert it into the stoma. If the doctor instructs, add this procedure to the list of care techniques that your patient should learn before leaving the hospital.

You'll know you've mastered peristomal care when you can prevent all urine leaks. The two main causes of such leaks are a poorly applied skin barrier (if you're using the ring type) and an improperly fitted faceplate. A poorly applied skin barrier has wrinkles in it, which allow urine to leak out and excoriate peristomal skin. Avoid this by practicing skin-barrier application until you're expert at it. An improperly fitted faceplate permits urine to pool around the stoma, causing skin excoriation. You can avoid this by adjusting the hole size in the faceplate or by acidifying the patient's urine. You can accomplish acidification by increasing your patient's intake of fluids containing vitamin C.

Your first indication of skin breakdown may be when the patient complains of a burning sensation under the faceplate. If this happens, begin treatment immediately. For mild skin excoriation, clean the area with warm water and let it dry. Then, dust the area lightly with karaya powder and spray or paint on a thin layer of protective dressing. Never use spray alone on irritated skin. Some hospitals recommend painting the irritated skin with an antacid (preferably the thick liquid that collects at the bottom of its container) before powdering and spraying the area.

If you're dealing with severe skin excoriation, you may be instructed to apply a Stomahesive® skin barrier. This not only protects the skin, but also encourages healing.

☎ *Nursing tip:* You can make the barrier adhere better to excoriated skin if you sprinkle karaya powder over the area first.

Has the excoriation persisted and become a pustular rash? If so, a yeast or fungal infection is responsible. In such a case, the doctor will probably want a culture and order application of nystatin powder or Kenalog* spray. He will not order creams or ointments since they can interfere with the faceplate's adhesion.

Help control odor by keeping the ostomy pouch clean. Do this by soaking it in detergents that contain deodorants. Or you can soak it in a solution that is one-part white vinegar and one-part water. Such a solution may also be used to treat alkaline incrustation on the faceplate or to treat skin excoriation. After the pouch dries, dust it with cornstarch.

The doctor may also order oral medication or special deodorizing substances placed directly in the pouch to minimize odor.

*Available in both the United States and in Canada

Ostomy management

Applying a disposable ostomy pouch

1 *Your patient's recovering from ileal conduit surgery, which he underwent 5 days ago. When you enter his room, you see that urine is leaking from around the faceplate of his disposable ostomy pouch. Do you know how to replace the faceplate and pouch with new ones? Follow this procedure:*

You'll need a disposable pouch, (such as the Nu-Hope adult postop pouch with adhesive-backed faceplate, which we're featuring here), an ostomy pouch belt, a liquid skin barrier (such as the Skin-Prep wipes featured here), gauze pads, a stoma guide, an adhesive solvent, and not shown, clean examining gloves, rubber band, and a safety pin.

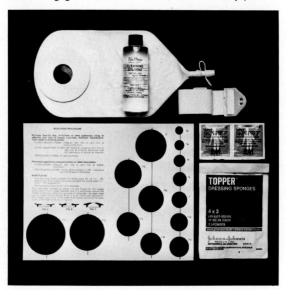

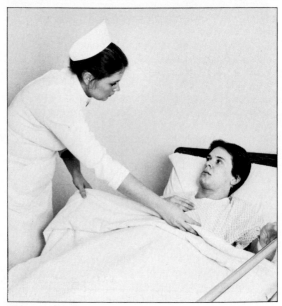

2 Make sure the patient's room is warm and well lighted. As you position the patient flat on his back, explain the procedure to him. Wash your hands. Then, put on clean examining gloves.

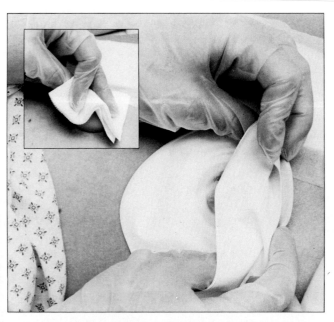

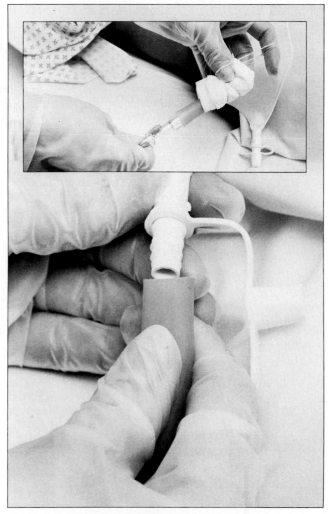

3 Remove the patient's old pouch by grasping the pouch and gently pulling it away from his skin. If it doesn't pull away easily, loosen the seal with warm water, or, if necessary, adhesive solvent. Then, use the stoma guide to make sure you have the correct size faceplate.

[Inset] Place a gauze pad over the stoma to absorb any urine leakage. If the pad gets saturated, replace it with a fresh one.

4 Disconnect the old pouch from the collection bag that's attached to the bed frame. Cover the collection bag tubing with a gauze pad and rubber band, as the nurse is doing in the inset, and secure it to the bed with a safety pin.

5 Gently wash the peristomal area with warm water and let it dry. Don't rub the area or you'll irritate the skin.
   Now, you're ready to apply the skin barrier. Cover the stoma with a rolled gauze pad to protect it. Then, in a circular motion, wipe Skin-Prep around the stoma. Let it dry for 30 seconds.

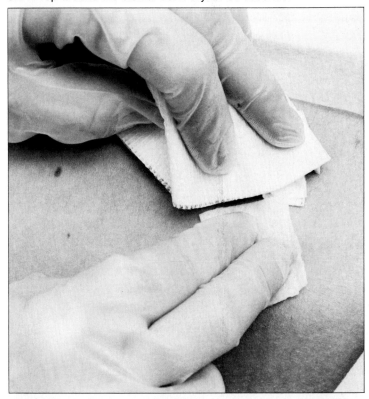

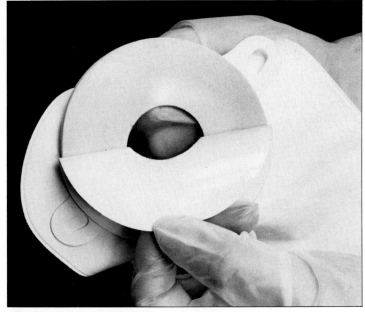

6 Now you're ready to apply the pouch. Begin by removing the paper backing from the foam pad on the faceplate, as the nurse is doing here.

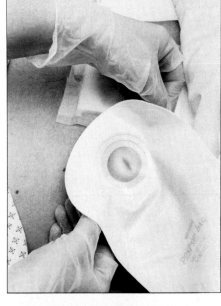

7 Then, center the faceplate over the stoma and gently press down on it. *Important:* Do not wrinkle the seal because doing so will allow leakage.

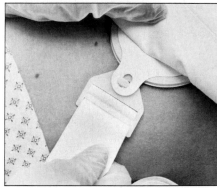

8 Hook the belt onto one side of the faceplate. Bring the belt around your patient's waist and hook the other end to the faceplate. Adjust the belt so it fits snugly.

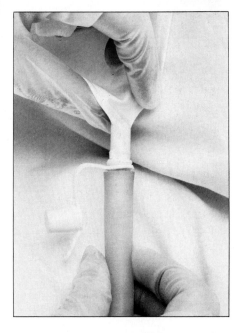

9 Now, unpin the collection-bag tubing, remove the rubber band and the gauze pad, and connect the tubing to the end of the pouch. Remember to document the procedure in your nurses' notes.

Ostomy management

Using a ring-type skin barrier

1 *Suppose you're not using a liquid skin barrier like the one featured in the preceding photostory. Then you'll use a ring that needs to be moistened or a ring that's adhesive backed.*

If you're using a ring that needs moistening, apply it in this way: First, measure the patient's stoma using the stoma guide.

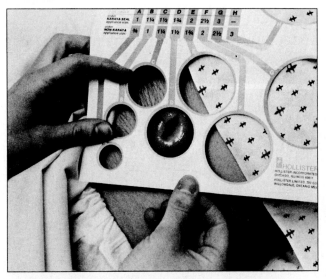

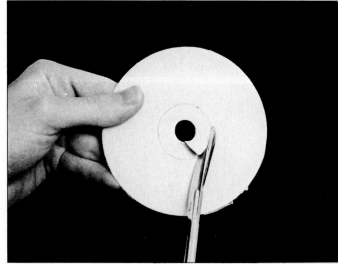

2 Next, select the correct size ring or cut the ring to size. Then, moisten it with warm water and rub it until it's sticky.

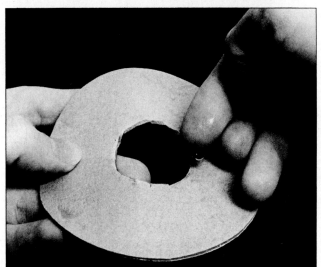

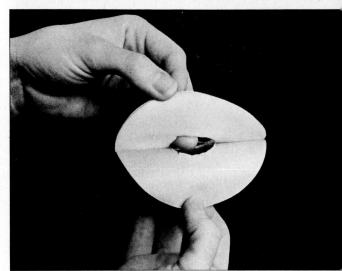

3 Center the ring over your patient's stoma and gently press the ring to the skin.

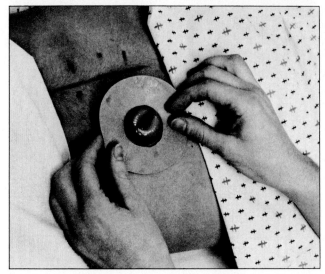

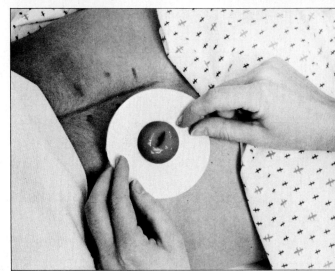

4 If you're using a ring that's adhesive backed, apply it in this way: Measure the patient's stoma, using the stoma guide. Select the correct size ring or cut one to size.

5 Then, remove the paper backing from the ring, to expose the adhesive.

6 Place the ring, adhesive side down, around the stoma. Press it gently to the skin. Now you're ready to apply the faceplate and pouch, following the procedure detailed in the preceding photostory.

Catheterizing an ileal conduit

1 *Henry Coleman, a 23-year-old government employee, is recovering from ileal conduit surgery. His doctor has instructed you to take a urine specimen. You know that you can't aspirate the specimen from Mr. Coleman's collection bag because the specimen won't be sterile. You have to catheterize him, but do you know how?*

Begin the procedure by getting a straight-catheter care kit (which includes a No. 14 or 16 French Robinson catheter, plastic-coated drape, precut drape, povidone-iodine solution, urine specimen cup, cotton balls, forceps, water-soluble lubricating jelly, graduated container, and sterile gloves), and a 4"x4" sterile gauze pad (not shown).

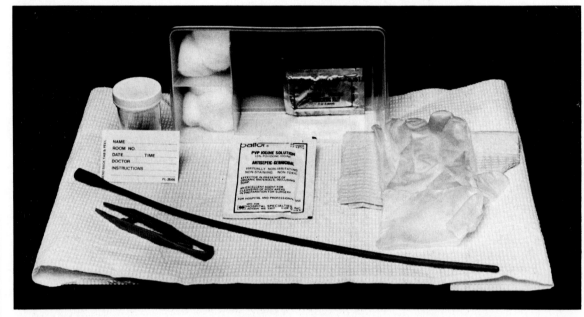

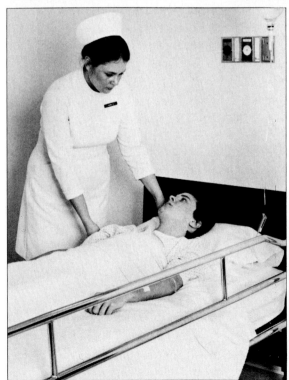

2 Explain the procedure to the patient. Answer any questions he may have before proceeding.

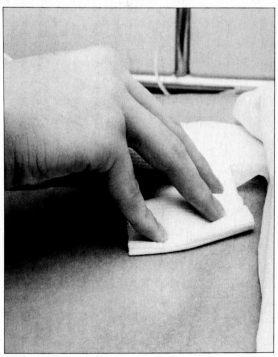

3 Remove the patient's ostomy pouch. Take the 4"x4" sterile gauze pad and ask Mr. Coleman to hold it intermittently against his stoma to absorb any urine that drains prior to catheterization.

Ostomy management

Catheterizing an ileal conduit continued

4 Put on sterile gloves and, observing sterile technique, place the precut drape around the stoma.

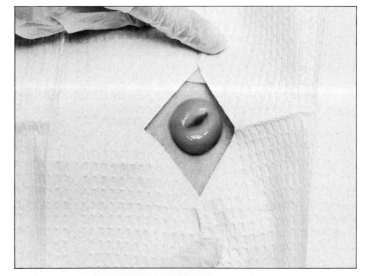

5 Prep the peristomal area with povidone-iodine solution.

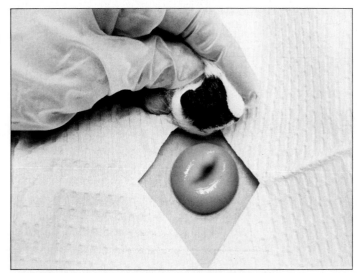

6 Open the lubricant packet. Insert the tip of the Robinson catheter into the packet and lubricate it.

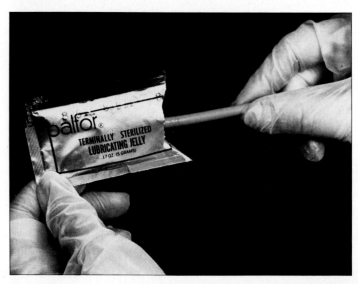

7 Insert the catheter into the stoma about 3″.

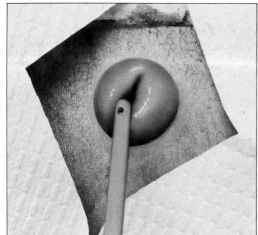

8 Allow urine to drain into the specimen cup; then drain the remaining urine into a graduated container. Pinch the catheter closed and remove it. Cap the specimen and reapply the pouch. Label the specimen and send it to the lab. Finally, document the procedure in your nurses' notes.

Dealing with ostomy complications

When you're caring for any patient, one of your most important goals is preventing complications. That's particularly true for the postsurgical patient. Of course, the best way to avoid complications is to provide the patient with meticulous and complete postop care. Turn to pages 78 and 79 to refresh yourself on the fundamentals of this care.

But when complications occur, you can minimize them if you recognize their signs and symptoms and notify the doctor immediately. For example, your patient may experience a fluid and electrolyte imbalance. We've detailed on page 80 how you can identify a fluid and electrolyte imbalance. To learn about other common ostomy complications and what to do about them, read this chart.

Complication	Signs and symptoms	Nursing action
Wound infection	• Elevated temperature • Purulent, malodorous drainage • Reddened, swollen, hard incision • Pain at incision • Elevated white-blood-cell count	• Maintain strict aseptic technique during dressing change. • Take wound culture. • Take patient's temperature every 4 hours until it stays normal for at least 48 hours. • Apply warm soaks to the incision, as ordered. • Force fluids, if not contraindicated. • Give antibiotics, antipyretics, and pain medication, as ordered. • Take special wound and skin precautions, as your hospital policy dictates. (See the NURSING PHOTOBOOK CONTROLLING INFECTION for more details.)
Intestinal obstruction	• No drainage from NG tube • Sharp, colicky pain in abdomen • Constipation or no bowel movement • Abdominal distention • Nausea and vomiting • Increased peristalsis above obstruction and no bowel sounds below obstruction • Diarrhea, if obstruction is partial or incomplete	• Insert a nasogastric tube to suction, as ordered. • Administer medication, such as Prostigmin*, to relieve gas, as ordered. • Insert rectal tube to relieve distention. • Administer fluids and electrolytes, as ordered. • Give patient nothing by mouth. • Ambulate the patient unless contraindicated by the doctor. • Prepare the patient for surgery, if the doctor orders.
Stenosis of the stoma	• Little or no urinary drainage • Pain around stoma	• Dilate stoma, using a graduated stylet or a catheter, as ordered. • Prepare the patient for surgery, if the doctor must reconstruct the stoma.
Dehiscence (partial or complete separation of wound) Evisceration (extrusion of internal organs through incision)	• Patient complains of pulling or "giving" of incision. • Excessive clear or serosanguineous fluid leakage from incision • Visual confirmation of complication	• Patient should lie flat with knees bent to relieve abdominal tension. • Caution patient not to cough or put undue strain on his incision if at all possible. • Don't give patient anything to eat or drink. • Apply warm, sterile dressings soaked in saline solution over incision and/or protruding intestines to prevent mucous membranes of intestines from drying out. • Take vital signs. • Observe for signs of shock. • Start an I.V. infusion, as ordered. • Notify doctor. He'll probably suture the wound, after administering local anesthesia. • To prevent dehiscence or evisceration, apply binder to abdomen of an elderly or diabetic patient, a patient with poor nutritional status, or a patient with pendulous abdomen.

*Available in both the United States and in Canada

Ostomy management

Rehabilitating the ostomate

You and your patient have conquered the first step of ostomy rehabilitation when he can look at his stoma. Achieving this initial level of acceptance is essential before you can begin patient teaching.

When you think he's ready, ask the patient to watch you empty his pouch. Eventually, instruct him in the procedure and ask him to help you. Use the home care aid on pages 104 and 105 to teach the patient each step. By the time he leaves the hospital, he should be capable of caring independently for his ostomy.

Your patient may not accept his stoma during his hospital stay. He may never accept it. But, there are several ways you can help him toward achieving this goal.

Begin by having the patient dress in his favorite outfit and stand before a full-length mirror. Realizing that he can hardly detect the ostomy under his clothes may in itself give him an optimistic outlook.

In most cases, he won't need to alter his clothing to accommodate an ostomy pouch. Tight undergarments and tight pants are the only articles of clothing that you should discourage your patient from wearing. A male ostomate should wear briefs. He may choose to wear suspenders instead of a belt, but, depending on stoma placement, this is not always necessary.

If a female ostomate wants to wear a girdle, instruct her to wear a lightweight one. Also, inform her that she can wear a two-piece swimsuit if it isn't too revealing.

Assure the patient that he can return to his job. However, if the job involves heavy lifting, instruct him to talk to the doctor before resuming it.

Tell your patient that he can resume almost all his former activities unless, of course, other physical problems contra-indicate this. The ostomate can participate in sports such as golf, tennis, skiing, scuba diving, and skydiving. However, if he wishes to participate in these sports, he should first reinforce the seal on his faceplate. Warn him to avoid strenuous body-contact sports, such as wrestling and football.

Inform your patient that he can eat almost anything he wants. However, he should avoid foods that affect urine odor, such as asparagus. The doctor may encourage the patient to increase fluid intake, particularly those fluids high in vitamin C.

Tell the female ostomate that pregnancy will cause no special problems for her. But, urge her to discuss the matter with her doctor before she becomes pregnant.

Remind the ostomy patient that, if he travels, he should carry an extra pouch, faceplate, and cleaning materials with him at all times, but not packed away in his luggage. This way, if his luggage gets lost or is temporarily inaccessible, he won't have problems.

Is your patient a child? Involve his parents in the child's rehabilitation. Urge them not to feel embarrassed about their child's stoma or try to conceal it. Instruct them not to limit their child's activities any more than they usually would. The more objectively they treat their child's condition, the quicker and easier he'll adjust to it.

No matter how carefully you teach your patient, you may never know whether or not he reaches the final goal: total acceptance of the ostomy as part of his body. However, you can get him started toward that goal by following the steps you've learned here.

Easing your patient's sexual adjustment

You can't consider your patient's postop rehabilitation complete unless he makes a good sexual adjustment. He'll have to be at ease with his new body image before he can hope for a satisfying sex life. Depending on the nature of his ostomy surgery, he may also have organic sexual difficulties. In either case, you can help.

The doctor will discuss sexual readjustment with the patient or ask you to. If the patient's too embarrassed or seems ashamed to discuss the subject, consider calling in someone who specializes in sexual counseling. Agencies such as the United Ostomy Association or the American Cancer Society can help put a new ostomate at ease. They can also provide helpful literature on the subject, if you think it would help.

Is the ostomate married? Suggest counseling for his spouse, if it seems appropriate. If the ostomate is single, encourage him to tell his partner about his ostomy soon after he returns home. This will prevent misunderstandings and feelings of embarrassment later.

An impotent male patient may be interested in penile implant surgery. If he is, arrange for a doctor to discuss the possibility with him. If you'd like to learn about penile implant surgery, see pages 86 and 87.

see pages 86 and 87.

PATIENT TEACHING

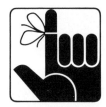

Teaching self-care to the ostomy patient

If you're preparing an ostomy patient to care for himself at home, you'll have to teach him general ostomy care, as well as one of these two techniques: applying a reusable pouch, or performing continent-vesicostomy self-catheterization.

For a guide to general ostomy care, copy the home care aid on the right and give it to your patient. Urge him to follow the instructions carefully.

If your patient's going home with a reusable ostomy pouch, make a copy of the home care aid on pages 104 and 105, and give it to him. Since application procedures differ, depending on the type of pouch your patient's using, modify the instructions to suit his particular needs. Then, go over the procedure several times to make sure he's doing it correctly.

If a more detailed discussion of reusable pouch application will help you, refer to the NURSING PHOTOBOOK PERFORMING GI PROCEDURES.

Does your patient have a continent vesicostomy? He'll go home with a suprapubic catheter in his bladder for irrigation and a straight catheter in his stoma acting as a stent. Teach him how to irrigate his suprapubic catheter with a bulb syringe. To do this, the patient should fill the bulb syringe with about 30 ml normal saline solution once each day and instill the solution into his suprapubic catheter. The solution should return spontaneously. If it doesn't, show the patient how to use the syringe bulb to gently suction the fluid from his bladder. If this technique doesn't work, tell the patient to call his doctor.

Instruct the patient to return to the hospital after 1 month so the doctor can remove both tubes. After removal, your patient must learn how to drain urine from his bladder using self-catheterization. The home care aid on the right is designed to help you teach him this technique. Copy it for him and review the procedure together. Then, watch him catheterize himself to make sure he's doing it correctly.

Patient teaching

Home care

Ostomy care: Tips and reminders

Dear Patient:

Your enterostomal therapist or nurse has taught you how to care for your stoma and pouch when you go home. Here's a list of some other things you should know:

• Call your doctor if your temperature rises to 101° F. (38.3° C.) or more.

• If you become constipated, take a mild laxative. If the problem continues, tell your doctor at your next appointment.

• If you develop diarrhea, call your doctor. He'll probably tell you to take Kaopectate® or Pepto-Bismol®.

• Don't lift objects heavier than a folding chair for at least 4 weeks after surgery, as you will not be completely healed.

• Don't drive or ride in a car unnecessarily for 4 weeks. A sudden stop could strain your abdominal muscles.

• Each day, clean the area around your stoma. Doing so is important because mucus collects and can cause irritation. During cleaning, check your stoma to make sure it's as pink and moist as the inside of your cheek. Report any change, such as black spots, to your doctor.

• You may notice a slight bulging to one side of your stoma. Don't become alarmed. This can result from a weakness in the abdominal muscles. Notify your doctor at your next appointment.

• Drink ____ to ____ 8-oz. glasses of water daily to help your urinary tract function properly. If your urine output seems scanty or stops completely, call your doctor immediately.

• If the skin around your stoma becomes red or sore, the area's probably been irritated by urine. You can prevent or correct this by keeping the area clean and dry and by applying your ostomy pouch carefully.

• Always carry an extra pouch and faceplate in your car when you're out, in case your faceplate comes loose.

With practice, you'll find that caring for your ostomy and pouch is easy. Then, as you gain confidence in your ability, your lifestyle will become more normal.

Home care

How to catheterize your continent vesicostomy

Dear Patient:

The nurse has shown you how to catheterize your continent vesicostomy. This home care aid is designed to remind you of each step.

• Begin by gathering this equipment and placing it on a clean towel: a red rubber catheter, lubricant, a povidone-iodine skin wipe, a 4"x4" sterile gauze pad, paper tape or any nonallergenic tape, and a container for collecting urine.

Note: You'll need a sterile container if the doctor wants to use your urine specimen for laboratory analysis.

• Open the lubricant packet. Insert about 3" of the catheter into the packet to lubricate the tip for easier insertion.

• Then, remove the gauze pad covering your stoma. Discard the pad. Clean the stoma and the area around it with the povidone-iodine wipe. Do this by starting at the stoma and working outward in a circular motion.

• Gently insert the catheter into the stoma. Urine will begin to flow. When the flow stops, pinch the catheter closed and remove it.

• Dry the skin, if necessary. Apply and tape a fresh sterile gauze pad over your stoma to keep it clean.

You may reuse your catheter, but first you must sterilize it. To do this, first immerse it in boiling water for 3 minutes. Then, to store it, wrap it in foil or place it in a plastic bag.

Patient teaching

Home care

Applying a reusable pouch

1 Dear Patient:
The nurse has taught you how to apply a reusable ostomy pouch. This home care aid is designed to remind you of each step.

Begin by gathering this equipment: a reusable pouch, faceplate and O-ring, a double-sided adhesive foam pad, gauze pads, and a skin barrier. (You'll also need scissors, if you're using a skin barrier that must be cut to size.)

Drain the urine from your pouch. Wash your hands.

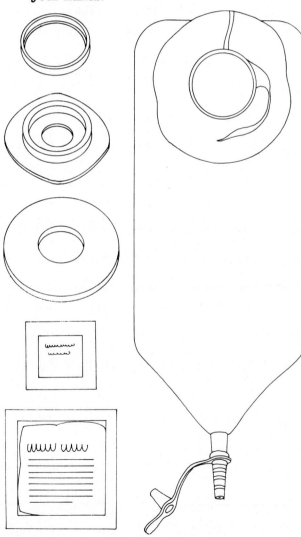

2 Lay the clean pouch on a flat surface, with the cup facing up. Slip the O-ring around the cup, with the O-ring's protruding edge against the pouch. Then, fold the cup down over the ring.

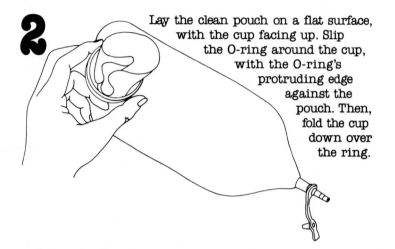

3 Firmly press the faceplate against the ring. Snap them together to provide a tight seal.

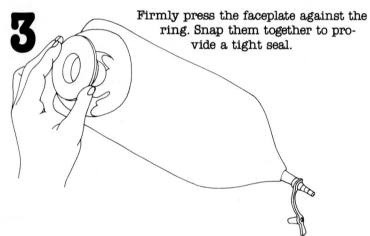

4 Peel off the paper backing from one side of the double-sided adhesive disc. Center the disc, sticky side down, over the faceplate. Firmly press the disc onto the faceplate.

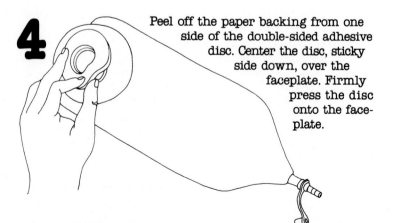

5 Remove the old pouch. If necessary, use warm water to loosen the adhesive. Then, set the pouch aside for later cleaning.

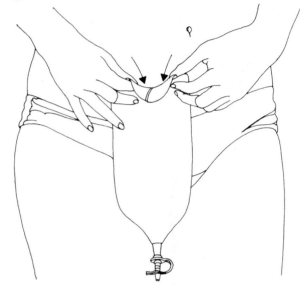

6 Cover the stoma with a rolled gauze pad to absorb any leaking urine. Gently wash your stoma and peristomal area with warm water and pat the area dry. Don't rub the area dry or you'll irritate the skin.

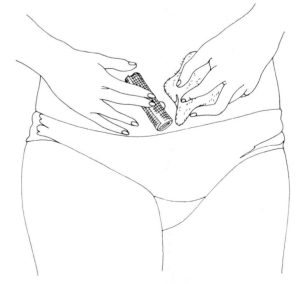

7 Now, still holding the rolled gauze pad over the stoma, apply the skin barrier of choice.

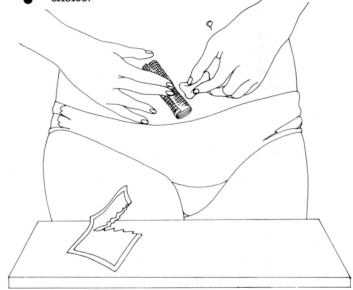

8 Now, remove the paper backing from the foam pad on the faceplate.
Center the faceplate over the stoma and gently press down on it. Make sure you don't wrinkle the seal. By carefully avoiding wrinkles, you'll prevent urine leakage.

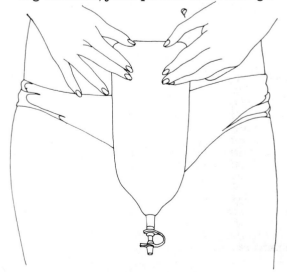

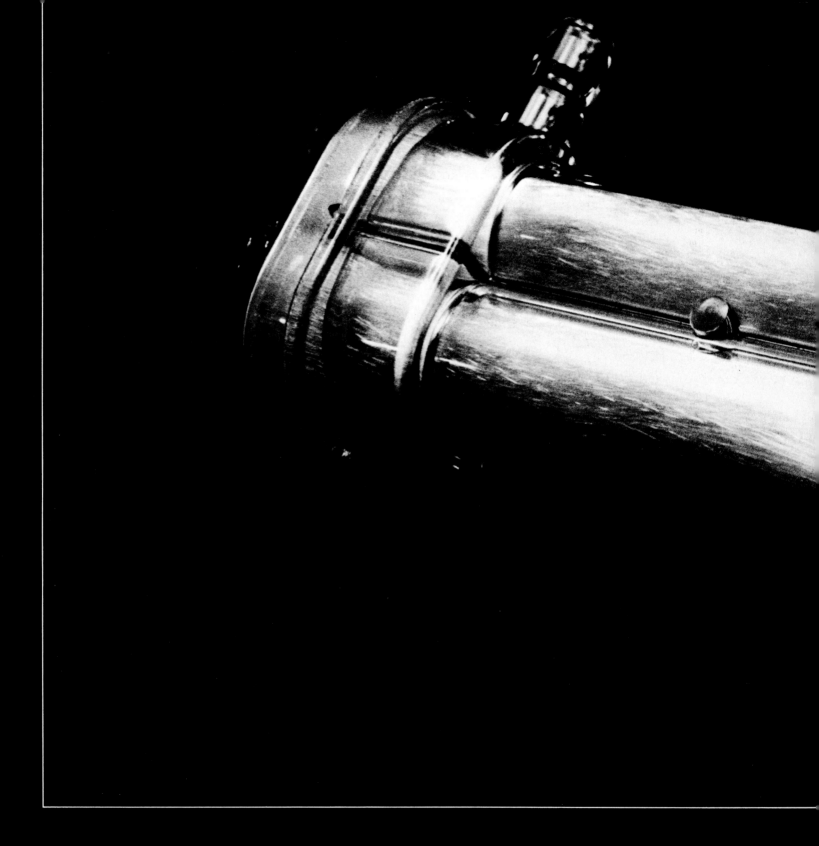

Caring for the Dialysis/Transplant Patient

Dialysis

Renal transplant

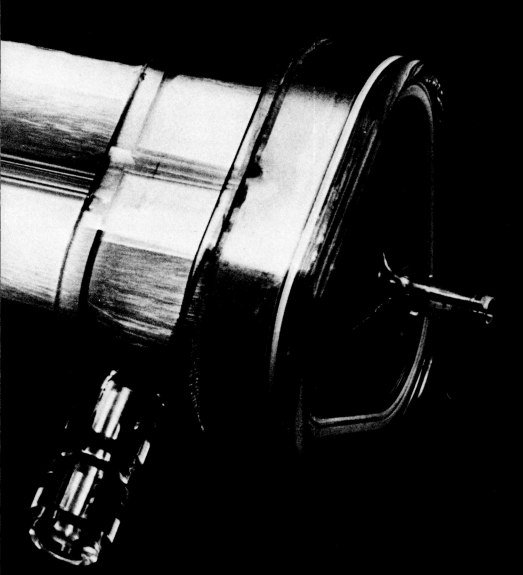

Dialysis

Thousands of people currently suffer from acute or chronic renal failure. Sooner or later you're likely to care for one of them. To do so, you need to know all about dialysis and renal transplant. Over the next few pages, we'll discuss renal failure basics and dialysis techniques. On pages 144 to 153, we'll explore renal transplant.

Put simply, the function of dialysis therapy is to clean the blood when the kidneys can't. The two methods of dialysis are called hemodialysis and peritoneal dialysis. Hemodialysis involves extracorporeal circulation, so the doctor must create an access to the patient's circulatory system. How do you care for the patient? Read the following pages to learn:
• how circulatory access is achieved.
• how to use different types of access to perform hemodialysis.
• how to care for the patient during hemodialysis.

To care for the patient receiving peritoneal dialysis, you'll perform one of two procedures, depending on whether your patient's in acute renal failure, or the last stage of chronic renal failure, called end stage renal disease (ESRD). We'll detail these procedures on the pages that follow.

If your ESRD patient is highly motivated, he may elect to receive continuous ambulatory peritoneal dialysis (CAPD). You'll find out how you can assist him in a CAPD program later in this section.

Learning about renal failure treatment

In renal failure, a patient's body accumulates wastes so rapidly that death is a certainty if the condition goes untreated. But, two treatments—dialysis and renal transplant—can prolong life for an indefinite period. In dialysis, the patient uses either a machine equipped with a semipermeable filtering membrane or his own peritoneal membrane to clean his blood. In renal transplant, the doctor surgically implants a healthy kidney from a compatible donor.

Dialysis can't cure renal failure, but merely approximates some renal functions. For example, dialysis conserves nutrients, regulates acid-base balance, and maintains fluid and electrolyte levels, though less efficiently than the kidney. Two functions it can't perform are secreting hormones and activating vitamin D.

In cases of acute renal failure, dialysis works well enough to substitute for the kidney until the kidney recovers. For the end stage renal disease (ESRD) patient, it may sustain life for years.

An alternative treatment for ESRD patients is renal transplant, with recipients and donors matched by careful tissue and blood typing. But, transplant surgery does not always prove successful because a patient's immune system may reject the donor's kidney as a foreign body. However, use of tissue-typing and immunosuppressive drugs has lowered the rejection rate. If the donor kidney is rejected, the patient must return to a dialysis therapy program. Depending on his condition and the availability of donor kidneys, a second transplant may or may not be attempted.

Nurses' guide to renal failure

Renal failure means that the kidneys no longer function properly. In acute renal failure, the kidneys reduce urine output suddenly, causing immediate symptoms. In chronic renal failure, the kidneys lose their function gradually, over a period of months or years. The patient may be asymptomatic until the later stages. By the time symptoms appear, his condition may be irreversible. This chart compares acute and chronic renal failure.

Type	Possible cause
Acute	*Prerenal (outside of genito-urinary system):* • Dehydration • Circulatory collapse • Salt depletion *Renal (within kidney):* • Trauma; for example, a crushing injury • Postoperative shock and blood transfusion reaction • Ingestion of nephrotoxic substances; for example, heavy metals, or drugs such as phenacetin • Renal infarction • Bacterial infection of kidney, or septicemia from bacterial infection • Intrarenal precipitation, such as hypercalcemia *Postrenal (outside kidney but within genitourinary system):* • Obstruction in urinary tract; for example, from calculi, tumor, or prostatitis
Chronic	• Any sufficiently severe cause of renal dysfunction, such as glomerulonephritis, polycystic kidney disease, hypertension, nephrosclerosis, diabetes, obstruction, infection, salt or water depletion, and systemic lupus erythematosus

Clinical course	Prognosis
• During the first phase, called the *oliguric phase,* urine output suddenly decreases to less than 400 ml per day, with elevated blood urea nitrogen (BUN), serum creatinine, and potassium levels. This phase may last from a few days to more than a month. • During the second phase, called the *diuretic phase,* the urine output increases to more than 400 ml per day. It may be as high as 8 liters per day. BUN, serum creatinine, and potassium stabilize at elevated levels, then decrease, and eventually reach normal levels. This phase also may last from a few days to a month. If not reversed, patient's condition deteriorates to chronic renal failure.	• If caused by problem outside of genitourinary system, renal failure is reversible, provided it's treated early. • If caused by bacterial infection, drug reaction, or metabolic disorder, renal failure may be reversible. • If caused by obstruction in urinary tract, renal failure may be reversible if obstruction is removed before renal damage occurs.
• In the first stage, called the *diminished renal reserve stage,* renal tissue is destroyed, but patient remains asymptomatic. • In the second stage, called the *renal insufficiency stage,* the patient may exhibit elevated BUN and creatinine levels, but show only vague signs and symptoms, such as increased blood pressure, nocturia, lassitude, fatigue, and decreased mental acuity. However, the patient may also have more severe signs and symptoms, such as muscular hyperactivity and cramps; gastrointestinal disturbances, such as anorexia, nausea, diarrhea, or ammonia breath; or congestive heart failure. • In the third stage, called *end stage renal disease (ESRD),* the patient shows elevated BUN and serum creatinine levels; fluid and electrolyte level imbalances (including hyperkalemia); and worsening of all previously mentioned signs and symptoms. The patient may have additional gastrointestinal disturbances, such as hemorrhage. Also, you may detect tissue wasting, skin discoloration, pruritis or uremic frost, hypertension, cardiac arrhythmias, congestive heart failure, neuromuscular disorders, tetany, psychologic disturbances, blood dyscrasias, amenorrhea, decreased fertility in females, and impotence in males.	• Whether chronic renal failure can be retarded depends on the nature of the underlying disorder. Infection and obstruction, for example, may be controlled. But, chronic renal disorders, such as polycystic kidney disease and nephrosclerosis, usually don't respond well to treatment. Such conditions result in end stage renal disease (ESRD), in which the kidneys lose all or most of their function and can no longer support life without assistance.

Understanding dialysis

Almost every renal failure patient undergoes dialysis. The patient depends on this procedure to clean his blood until his kidneys recover or he receives a new kidney. Or, he may use dialysis for the rest of his life. In dialysis, waste particles and fluids move from the blood, across a semipermeable membrane, and into dialysate, the solution on the other side of the membrane. Then, the dialysate is drained away, removing the blood's waste products with it.

Three chemical principles govern dialysis: diffusion, osmosis, and ultrafiltration. *Diffusion* refers to the movement of particles through a semipermeable membrane, from the side of higher concentration to the side of lower concentration, until the particle concentrations become equal on both sides of the membrane. *Osmosis* refers to the movement of fluids through a semipermeable membrane, flowing from the side of lower concentration to the side of higher concentration of particles until the particle concentrations on both sides of the membrane are equal. *Ultrafiltration* refers to the movement of fluids under pressure through a semipermeable membrane, from the side of the membrane under higher pressure to the side of the membrane under lower pressure.

When a patient undergoes dialysis, the dialysate initially contains purified water and the major electrolytes in concentrations that approximate extracellular body fluid. Dextrose and supplements such as potassium may be added. Urea and waste electrolytes move from their area of highest concentration (the blood) to their area of lowest concentration (the dialysate). If dextrose and potassium are more concentrated in the dialysate than in the bloodstream, these substances will move in the opposite direction.

Note: Knowing this is important. If your patient's serum potassium level is low, the doctor can correct this condition by adding extra potassium to the dialysate.

Excess water, as you know, moves from the blood into the dialysate.

That's how dialysis works, in principle. Renal patients can choose one of two types of dialysis: hemodialysis or peritoneal dialysis. In hemodialysis, a sheet of cellophane serves as the semipermeable membrane in the dialyzer machine; plastic tubing carries the blood from the body to the membrane. In peritoneal dialysis, the patient's own peritoneal lining serves as the membrane. The peritoneal blood vessels carry blood to the membrane.

Excess water is removed differently in each of these types of dialysis. Hemodialysis uses ultrafiltration, or pressure, to remove water from the blood, whereas peritoneal dialysis uses osmosis. To accomplish osmosis, dextrose is added to the dialysate to give it a higher particle concentration than the blood.

The chart on the following page compares hemodialysis and peritoneal dialysis in detail.

Dialysis

Comparing hemodialysis and peritoneal dialysis

Treatment	Requirements	Indications	Contraindications	Advantages	Disadvantages
Hemodialysis	• Access to circulatory system • Dialysate • Hemodialysis machine • Dialyzer	Acute and chronic renal failure where peritoneal dialysis can't be used because of: • Hypercatabolic states • Hyperkalemia • Diaphragmatic leaks • Severe respiratory insufficiency • Large abdominal wounds with drains • Intra-abdominal cancer • Multiple abdominal adhesions • Diffusely infected abdominal wall. (If the patient is not already on a dialysis program, start him on hemodialysis rather than peritoneal dialysis.) • Critical volume excess (such as pulmonary edema), or pericardial friction rub, where all alternative therapies have been exhausted	• Cardiovascular disease • Severe blood-clotting disorders • Circulatory instability	• This method usually requires only three treatments per week. • Treatment period is usually short (3 to 6 hours). • Treatment is four to six times more efficient than peritoneal dialysis in removing low molecular weight substances from blood.	• Treatment requires access to circulatory system. • Treatment is expensive, necessitating special equipment and trained personnel. (Home care is less expensive.) • During treatment, 350 to 600 ml blood circulates extracorporeally, reducing blood volume so much that small children or patients with ischemic heart disease have difficulty tolerating the treatment. • Patients may require blood transfusions during or between treatments, which usually must be performed in a hospital or outpatient clinic. • Rapid shifts in fluid and electrolyte levels may cause dialysis disequilibrium syndrome.
Peritoneal dialysis	• Access to peritoneum • Bag or bottle of dialysate • Tubing • Dialysate delivery machine (optional)	Acute and chronic renal failure, where hemodialysis can't be used because of: • Severe blood-clotting disorders • Cardiovascular disease • Exhausted circulatory access sites • Inadequate veins (usually occurring in very young or old patients) • Atherosclerotic veins (in diabetic patients) • Patient refusal to receive blood transfusions	• Severe hypercatabolic states • Paralytic ileus with abdominal distention • Diaphragmatic leaks • Severe respiratory insufficiency • Large abdominal wounds with drains • Intra-abdominal cancer • Multiple abdominal adhesions • Diffusely infected abdominal wall, unless the patient is already on a peritoneal dialysis program	• No circulatory access is necessary. • Treatment is less expensive than hemodialysis. • During treatment, the patient has low risk of an immediate life-threatening event, such as severe hemorrhage. • Fluid and electrolyte level shifts are usually gradual. • Diabetic patients have less retinopathy than those receiving hemodialysis. • Treatment is more efficient than hemodialysis for removal of middle weight molecular substances.	• Acute or intermittent peritoneal dialysis treatment can take from 10 to 48 hours. • Depending on length of treatment, more than three treatments per week may be necessary. For continuous ambulatory peritoneal dialysis (CAPD), treatment continues 24 hours per day. • Risk of peritonitis is high. • Because much protein loss occurs across peritoneal membrane, the patient must be given protein-rich diet.

Understanding how blood moves through the hemodialysis system

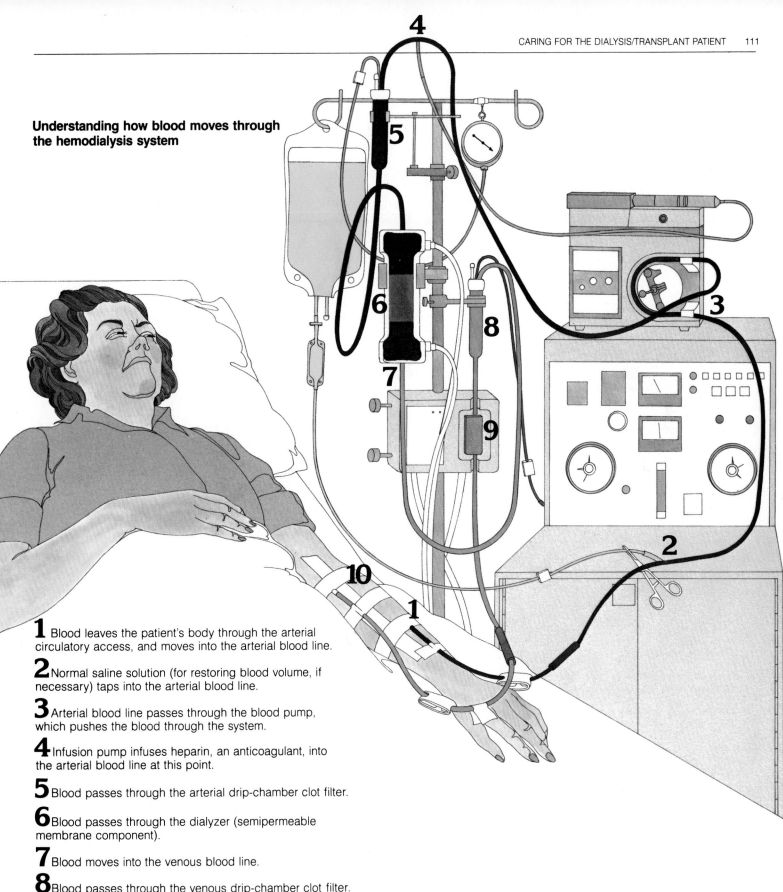

1 Blood leaves the patient's body through the arterial circulatory access, and moves into the arterial blood line.

2 Normal saline solution (for restoring blood volume, if necessary) taps into the arterial blood line.

3 Arterial blood line passes through the blood pump, which pushes the blood through the system.

4 Infusion pump infuses heparin, an anticoagulant, into the arterial blood line at this point.

5 Blood passes through the arterial drip-chamber clot filter.

6 Blood passes through the dialyzer (semipermeable membrane component).

7 Blood moves into the venous blood line.

8 Blood passes through the venous drip-chamber clot filter.

9 Blood passes through the air-foam detector.

10 Blood returns to the patient's body through the venous blood line and the venous circulatory access.

Dialysis

Learning about hemodialysis machines

Although hemodialysis machines come in a wide variety of models, they can be divided into two groups: negative-pressure and positive-pressure machines. Negative or positive refers to the direction of the pressure used for ultrafiltration.

Negative pressure
(See illustration to the right)

Dialyzer (semipermeable membrane component)
Flat plate or hollow fiber artificial kidney (HFAK) operates in a closed system, rather than in an open reservoir.

Ultrafiltration method
Negative pressure applied to the dialysate draws water from blood into dialysate.

Dialysate mixing system
• Often used with a proportioning mixing system. Dialysate concentrate is put in the machine, and the machine is connected to a water source. A proportioning pump automatically mixes the correct amounts of water and dialysate concentrate.

Nursing considerations
• Do not use a unipuncture machine (which alternately clamps arterial and venous blood lines) with a negative-pressure dialyzer. The unipuncture machine will allow too much pressure to build up in the dialyzer, which may rupture the semipermeable membrane.

Positive pressure

Dialyzer (semipermeable membrane component)
Coil set in open reservoir of dialysate

Ultrafiltration method
A Hoffman clamp on the venous blood line exerts positive pressure on the blood in the coil, forcing excess water from blood.

Dialysate mixing system
• Often used with a batch-tank mixing system. This system mixes enough dialysate (120 to 200 liters) for one treatment, using purified water and either dialysate concentrate or a mix of appropriate chemicals. Dialysate can be adjusted during treatment to meet patient's individual requirements.

Nursing considerations
• Positive pressure requires more blood outside of the body, which may cause hypovolemia in children or small adults.
• In spite of potential hypovolemia, for some patients positive pressure cleans the blood more effectively.

Identifying components of a negative-pressure hemodialysis machine

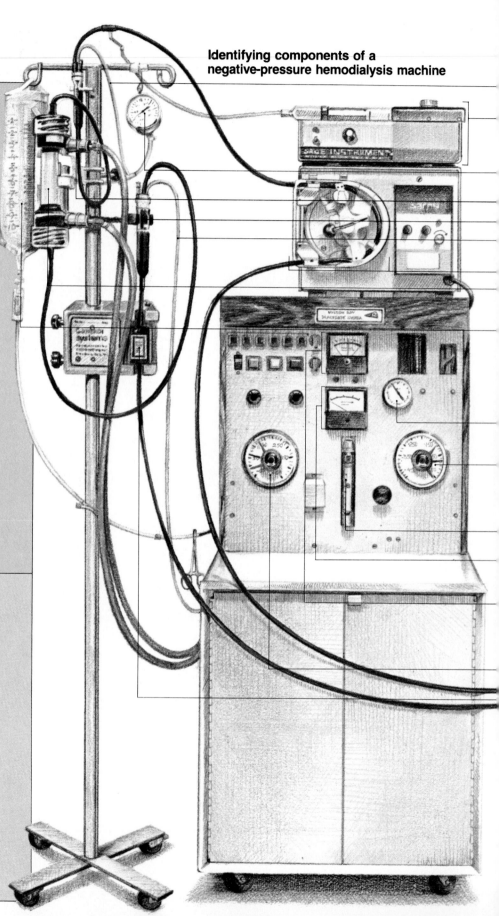

Pressure monitor line leads to arterial pressure gauge.

The infusion pump (optional) infuses heparin into the arterial tubing, for continuous heparinization. Or, minimal doses of heparin can be injected directly into the arterial blood line.

The arterial pressure gauge monitors pressure in arterial blood line.

The arterial drip chamber filters out blood clots.

The venous drip chamber filters out blood clots.

Pressure monitor line leads to venous pressure gauge.

The blood pump pushes blood through system.

The hollow fiber artificial kidney (HFAK) dialyzer permits fluid and waste transfer from the blood to the dialysate.

Heparinized normal saline solution is used to prime the dialyzer and blood lines. Then, the heparinized solution is replaced with a bag of nonheparinized normal saline solution. This solution helps retransfuse the blood at the end of a treatment. Or, it can be used to restore the patient's blood volume.

The temperature monitor indicates dialysate temperature. The monitor sounds an alarm if the temperature deviates from 37° C.

The pressure monitor helps determine the amount of fluid being removed from the patient's blood by ultrafiltration. The monitor sounds an alarm if the system does not maintain the preset pressure.

Dialysate flow regulator maintains flow rate at the preset level.

The blood leak detector sounds an alarm when a leak occurs in the semipermeable membrane.

The conductivity gauge monitors dialysate fluid. If dialysate's mixed improperly, an alarm sounds and the monitor cuts off the flow of dialysate. Should this happen, check the solution's chloride content and osmolality.

Venous pressure gauge indicates pressure of blood in venous line.

The air foam detector monitors the venous blood line for air bubbles in the patient's blood. If an air bubble's present, the monitor sounds an alarm and clamps the venous blood tubing to prevent the bubble from entering the patient's circulatory system.

Setting up proportioning negative-pressure hemodialysis equipment

Most patients requiring hemodialysis today use negative-pressure equipment, particularly those patients who are young or small. If you're caring for such a patient, here's how to set up and prime the negative-pressure equipment:
• First, attach the arterial and venous blood lines to the hemodialysis machine.
• Then, turn on the cold water faucet to allow treated water to enter the system.
• Turn on the hemodialysis machine.
• Check the dialysate concentrate jug in the machine to make sure it's filled with the solution prescribed by the doctor. Then, turn the machine to the dialyzer mode to activate the proportioning pump. The pump will begin combining dialysate and water. Check the indicator lights to make sure they're working. If any alarms sound, find out why. If the machine's monitors are defective, get new equipment.
• Now, fill two 20 cc flush syringes with normal saline solution from a 1,000 ml I.V. bag. Add 500 units heparin to each syringe. Set the syringes aside for use in preparing your patient's access site.
Note: If you're dialyzing with a single catheter or needle, fill only one 20 cc syringe.
• Next, inject 1,500 units heparin into the bag and insert an I.V. administration set spike into the bag. Hang the bag on the hemodialysis machine I.V. pole. Attach the I.V. tubing to the saline solution infusion T connector on the arterial blood line.
• Now, you're ready to prime the arterial line. To do so, unclamp the arterial line and allow saline solution to flow through the line into a bucket. Be careful not to touch the end of the arterial line to any part of the bucket. Clamp and cap the line and hang it on the machine.
• Now, you're ready to fill the arterial drip chamber. Turn on the blood pump. Unclamp the pressure monitor line so it's open to the arterial drip chamber. Allow the chamber to fill to three quarters full. Then, reclamp the line.
• To prime the remainder of the arterial line, unclamp the arterial line below the drip chamber. When the saline solution flows out the end of the arterial line, turn off the blood pump and reclamp the arterial line. Attach the line to the arterial blood port on the negative-pressure dialyzer.

• To prime the dialyzer, remove the clamp below the drip chamber. Then, turn on the blood pump. Allow saline solution to flow through the dialyzer. The saline solution will require about 3 minutes to reach the venous blood port. Before it reaches the port, you must attach the venous blood line to the port. Place the distal end of the line in the bucket, without letting it touch any part of the bucket. Clamp the end of the venous line.
• Now, you're ready to fill the venous drip chamber. Unclamp the pressure monitor line to the venous drip chamber. Allow the chamber to fill three quarters full. Then, clamp the line again.
• Next, unclamp the venous line. Allow 800 ml saline solution to run through the system into the bucket. Reclamp the line. Turn off blood pump.
• Now, run both dialysate and saline solution through the system. To do so, remove the cap from the end of the arterial line. Uncap the venous line and, using its cap fixture as a connector, connect the ends of both lines. Remove the clamps on the arterial and venous lines. Place a clamp on the saline solution infusion T, so no new saline solution can enter the system.
• Turn on the blood pump. Immediately attach the dialysate lines to the correct dialyzer inlet and outlet ports. *Note:* The dialysate flows countercurrent to the blood. Therefore, the inflow dialysate line connects to the port near the venous line and the outflow dialysate line connects to the port near the arterial line.
• Let the dialysate recirculate through the system, to wash out any foreign substances that may have been used to sterilize the dialyzer. After 5 minutes, turn off the blood pump. Then, clamp the arterial and venous lines. Disconnect the lines and cap them.
• Next, check the dialysate concentration to make sure it's isotonic to the blood. To determine this, check the chloride levels with a bedside chloride titration kit. Or, test the osmolality, using freezing-point depression test equipment or an osmolality meter. This step is very important, because use of a nonisotonic dialysate can cause death.
• Prepare your patient's access site, using the 20 cc syringes you filled earlier with heparinized saline solution.

Dialysis

Nurses' guide to hemodialysis access sites

Access	Insertion procedure	Indications	Advantages
Femoral vein catheterization 	Using the Seldinger technique, the doctor inserts an introducer needle into the right or left femoral vein. He then inserts a guide wire through the introducer needle and removes the needle. Using the guide wire, he threads a plastic or Teflon catheter, 5″ to 12″ long (12.7 to 30.5 cm), into the vein. The doctor may use a single catheter with a Y hub. Or, if he uses two catheters, he'll insert the second catheter for outflow, ½″ (1.3 cm) distal to the inflow catheter.	Acute or chronic renal failure	• Provides quick access to the circulatory system in emergencies.
Subclavian vein catheterization 	Using the Seldinger technique, the doctor inserts an introducer needle into the subclavian vein. He then inserts a guide wire through the introducer needle and removes the needle. Using the guide wire, he threads a 5″ to 12″ plastic or Teflon catheter (with Y hub) into the vein.	Acute or chronic renal failure	• Provides quick access to the circulatory system in emergencies. • Allows patient to move about freely. • Carries less risk of infection than femoral catheterization.
Arteriovenous (A-V) shunt 	The doctor makes an incision in the patient's wrist or ankle. Then, he inserts one 6″ to 10″ (15.2 to 25.4 cm) transparent Silastic cannula into an artery and another into a vein. He tunnels the cannulas out through stab wounds and connects them with a 1″ (2.5 cm) piece of Teflon tubing.	Acute or chronic renal failure in young or elderly patients with extremely small veins or a venous pattern too poor to allow vein grafts or fistulas.	• Provides arterial blood pressure for pumping blood. • Avoids repeated catheterization of patients with extended acute renal failure. • Permits hemodialysis without venipuncture for children or for adults who are afraid of needles.
Arteriovenous (A-V) fistula 	The doctor makes an incision in the patient's wrist. Then, he makes a small incision in the side of an artery and another incision in the side of a vein. He sutures the edges of these incisions together to create a common opening, 3 to 7 mm long.	Chronic renal failure	• Provides arterial blood pressure for pumping blood. • Carries minimal infection risk because fistula is subcutaneous. • Makes blood clotting less likely than with a shunt or graft, because the patient's own blood vessels are used. • Requires revision less frequently than shunt. • Doesn't restrict patient from using the affected arm or leg actively.
Arteriovenous (A-V) vein graft 	The doctor makes an incision in the patient's forearm, upper arm, or thigh. Then, he tunnels the natural or synthetic graft subcutaneously. He sutures the distal end of the graft to an artery. He sutures the proximal end to a vein.	Chronic renal failure in young or elderly patients with small arm veins or a venous pattern too poor for a fistula.	• Provides arterial blood pressure for pumping blood. • Doesn't restrict patient from using the grafted arm or leg actively.

Disadvantages	Nursing considerations	
• Catheter location immobilizes patient. • Bleeding may occur around catheter. • Severe hemorrhage may occur if catheter cap comes off. • Infection may occur. • Femoral artery may be punctured during insertion.	• Use for temporary access (average life: 1 week). • Begin hemodialysis immediately after insertion, to prevent blood clotting. • Usually, the catheter's used for only one hemodialysis treatment. But, the doctor may order it left in place for three such treatments. • After each hemodialysis treatment, flush the catheters,	and fill them with heparinized normal saline solution. Then, cap them and cover with a sterile dressing. • Don't permit patient to ambulate. Doing so may dislodge the catheter or damage the vein. • Don't permit patient to sit up in bed. Doing so may obstruct blood flow. Keep the head of the bed at a 45° angle.
• Bleeding may occur around catheter. • Severe hemorrhage may occur if catheter cap comes off. • Infection may occur. • Insertion may cause pneumothorax.	• Use for temporary access (average life: 1 to 2 weeks). • If a Y hub is used, also use unipuncture equipment, which alternately clamps arterial and venous tubing. • If the catheter is used only for outflow, insert an over-the-needle catheter into the patient's antecubital vein in the arm opposite the catheter, to accommodate venous return. • Begin hemodialysis immediately after insertion, to prevent clotting. • Usually, the catheter's used for only one hemodialysis treatment. But, the doctor may order it left in place for 3 to 6 dialyses.	• After each hemodialysis treatment, flush the catheter, and fill it with heparinized saline solution. Then, cap it with an injection cap and cover it with a sterile dressing. • Doctor will order a chest X-ray after each insertion, to rule out pneumothorax. • Cannot be used in patients with pulmonary hypertension.
• Patient must restrict activity in affected arm or leg. • Because shunt's a foreign body, clotting and infection risks are high. • Opening shunt for hemodialysis increases infection risk. • Shunt may accidentally separate, which can cause severe hemorrhage or death. Or, patient can easily separate shunt to commit suicide.	• Use for temporary or permanent access (average life: 7 to 10 months, sometimes longer). • For a few hours after insertion, have patient keep his arm or leg straight and elevated. If the shunt's in his leg, he'll need to use crutches for 3 weeks. Instruct the patient to keep his arm or leg as straight as possible at all times. • Change dressings as often as needed. • Monitor the shunt site frequently for good arterial flow. Palpate for thrill. Listen with a stethoscope for bruit. • Check the shunt site frequently for infection signs. • Control any severe bleeding with clamps or a tourniquet. Notify the doctor immediately.	• Check the blood color in shunt. (See chart on page 121 for details.) • Instruct patient to keep shunt clean and dry. Permit no bathing for 2 to 3 weeks after insertion. Then, tell the patient to protect the shunt with plastic while bathing. • Caution the patient to restrict activity in the affected arm or leg. Don't permit him to lift heavy objects. • Don't use the affected arm or leg for blood pressure readings or venipunctures. • Don't permit patient to wear constrictive jewelry or clothing over shunt site.
• Can't be used in a patient with small veins. • Blood clotting may occasionally occur if patient is severely dehydrated or hypotensive. • Atherosclerotic or diabetic patients may develop numbness, tingling, and coldness below fistula site from arterial insufficiency (steal syndrome).	• Use for permanent access (average life: 3 to 4 years). • Immediately after fistula surgery, keep the arm elevated. • Remove the dressings after 2 days, and clean the suture line with povidone-iodine solution. Apply new sterile dressings daily for 10 to 14 days, until sutures are removed. • Fistula may require 6 weeks to fully mature, so that the blood vessels are enlarged and their walls are thickened. But, if necessary, you may perform hemodialysis within 1 week postop. • Check the fistula periodically for good arterial blood flow; palpate the site for thrill; listen with a stethoscope for bruit.	• After you begin using the fistula for hemodialysis, scabs will form at the venipuncture site. Since these provide protection against infection, don't permit patient to pick at them or irritate them. However, you may use a skin-softening cream around the scabs. Cover large scabs with an adhesive bandage strip. • Wash the affected arm daily with antibacterial soap. • Do not use the affected arm for blood pressure readings or venipunctures (except when performing hemodialysis). • Don't permit patient to wear constrictive jewelry or clothing over the fistula site.
• Hypotension or mechanical obstruction, such as kinking, may cause clotting. • The tissues surrounding the graft may become infected easily, because the graft is a foreign body. • Atherosclerotic or diabetic patients may develop numbness, tingling, and coldness below fistula site from arterial insufficiency (steal syndrome).	• Use for permanent access (average life: 2 years). • Immediately after graft implantation, keep the arm or leg elevated. • Remove the dressings after 2 days, and clean the suture line with povidone-iodine solution. Apply new sterile dressings daily for 10 to 14 days, until sutures are removed. • Don't permit patient to wear constrictive jewelry or clothing over the graft site. • To prolong graft life, perform venipuncture using a single-needle double-lumen catheter. • Wash grafted arm or leg daily with antibacterial soap.	• Check graft several times daily for abnormal bruit and thrill, which indicate clotting. • After you begin using the graft for hemodialysis, scabs will form at the venipuncture site. Since these provide protection against infection, don't permit the patient to pick at them or irritate them. However, you may use a skin-softening cream around the scabs. • Don't use the arm with the graft for blood pressure readings or venipunctures (except when performing hemodialysis).

Dialysis

Performing daily arteriovenous shunt care

Because an arteriovenous (A-V) shunt extends the circulatory system outside of a patient's body, it requires daily care and observation. If each day you care properly for the shunt, you can prevent or minimize three major shunt problems: infection, clotting, or hemorrhage resulting from separation. By avoiding these problems, you can prolong shunt life and postpone the need for moving the shunt to a new site (shunt revision).

• To perform daily shunt care, obtain clean examining gloves, povidone-iodine solution, sterile 4"x4" gauze pads, sterile cotton-tipped applicators, povidone-iodine ointment, nonallergenic tape, elastic bandage, and scissors. Remember to wash your hands.

• Remove the patient's elastic bandage. Unclamp the bulldog clamps that are always attached to the dressing in case of emergency. Remove any gauze dressings covering the shunt. Check the area around the shunt for purulent drainage, redness, or extrusion of the Silastic tubing.

• Check the blood flow. To do this properly, first note blood color and temperature. (For details on how to assess blood color, see the chart on page 121.) Then, use a stethoscope between the arterial and venous cannula exit sites to confirm that blood's flowing at the proper rate.

• Put on the gloves. To clean the shunt site, soak the gauze pads with povidone-iodine solution. Then, beginning at the middle of the shunt, thoroughly clean the skin on one side of the shunt. Use a new pad for each stroke, and don't overlap the strokes.

• Use cotton-tipped applicators to gently remove any incrustations around the cannula on the side of the shunt you're cleaning. Change applicators frequently. Then, using clean pads and applicators, repeat the entire cleaning procedure on the other side of the shunt.

• Now, soak a gauze pad in povidone-iodine solution and gently clean the Silastic tubing of the connected cannulas.

• Use more soaked pads to clean that part of the skin that was covered by the elastic bandage. Dry the site thoroughly with gauze pads. Use a clean pad on each side of the shunt to avoid cross contamination.

• To provide additional protection against infection, apply povidone-iodine ointment around the cannula exit sites. *Important:* Discontinue use of this ointment if the patient's allergic to it.

• Next, tape the junction of the arterial and venous cannulas with nonallergenic tape to help prevent accidental separation.

• Cut a gauze pad to fit tightly around each cannula. Gently insert another gauze pad underneath the Silastic tubing of the connected cannulas, to cushion it.

• Finally, cover the shunt with another gauze pad and rewrap the site with the new elastic bandage. Check for tightness to make sure you don't impair blood circulation.

Performing hemodialysis using an arteriovenous shunt

1 *Because the risks of infection, clotting, and hemorrhage are higher with an arteriovenous (A-V) shunt, many doctors prefer to create fistulas or vein grafts. But, you still may encounter a patient with a shunt in place. If you do, will you know how to perform hemodialysis?*

To prepare for the procedure, first assemble the sterile equipment shown here: three drapes and a shunt-care tray, including gloves, 4"x4" gauze pads, two bulldog clamps, 20cc syringe, stainless steel cup, two shunt adapters, and test tubes.

In addition, obtain povidone-iodine solution, nonallergenic tape, 1,500 units of heparin (1,000 unit/ml), and a 250 ml bag of normal saline solution. For drawing heparin, obtain a 5cc syringe with a 21G, ⅝" needle (not shown).

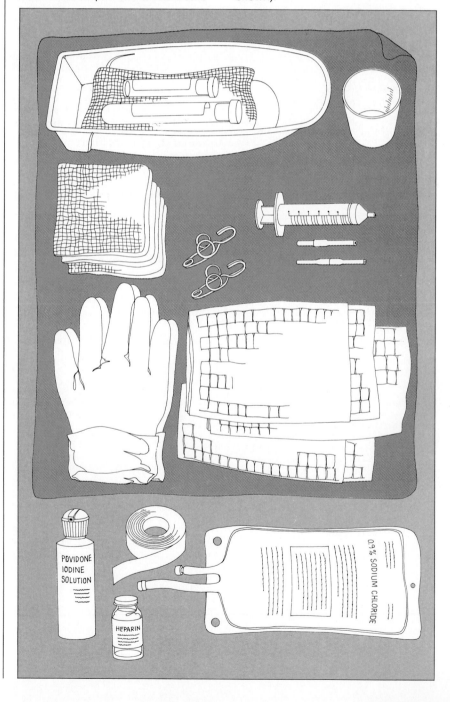

2 Explain the procedure to your patient. Then, weigh her, and take her vital signs. Take her blood pressure when she's standing up and lying down. Record this information on her hemodialysis record. Remember to wash your hands.

Place a bed-saver pad under the limb with the shunt. Perform daily care, as instructed on page 116, but don't reapply a clean dressing over the shunt.

You may work from a bedside table or you may place your equipment on the patient's bed. If you work from her bed, first place one drape on the bed, as shown here.

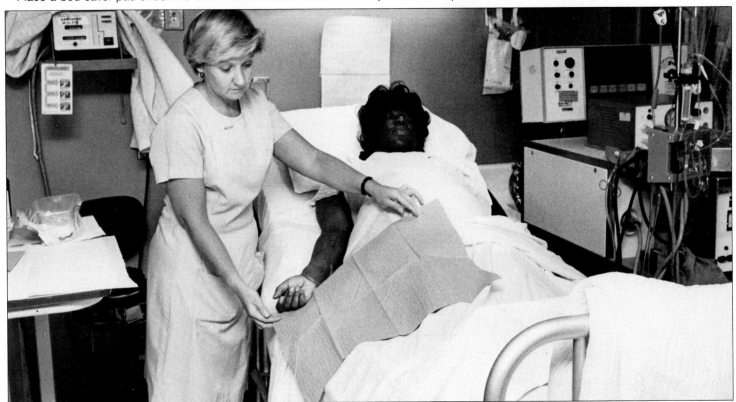

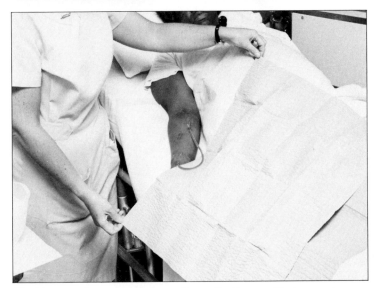

3 Now, you're ready to drape the patient's arm. To do so, place a drape on top of her lower arm, just below the shunt's arterial exit site.

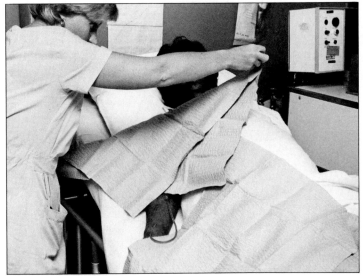

4 Then, fold a second drape, as shown, and use it to drape the patient's upper arm above the shunt's venous exit site.

Open the shunt-care kit aseptically, being careful not to touch the contents. Pour 300 ml saline solution into the cup in the kit tray. Add 1,500 units heparin. Now, put on the sterile gloves.

Dialysis

Performing hemodialysis using an arteriovenous shunt continued

5 To keep the shunt from coming into contact with the patient's skin, place gauze pads on the skin between the cannula exit sites. Use four pads in all, arranged as shown in the inset. Now, fill a 20 cc syringe with heparinized saline solution.

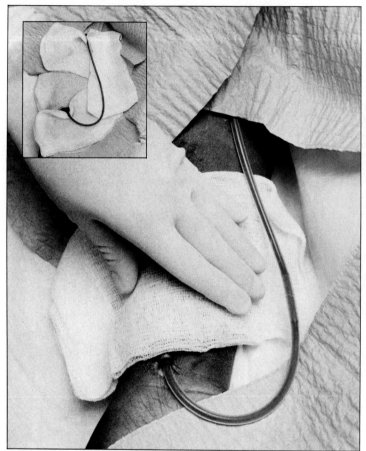

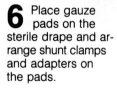

6 Place gauze pads on the sterile drape and arrange shunt clamps and adapters on the pads.

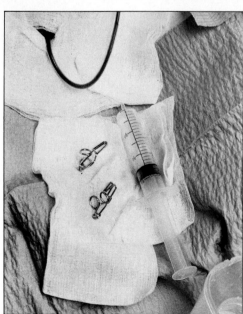

7 Prepare to separate the shunt cannulas by clamping both cannulas with bulldog clamps, applied about 2″ (5 cm) from the cannula junction.

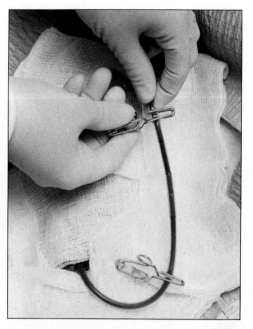

8 Separate the shunt cannulas. Leave the Teflon cannula connector in the end of one of the cannulas. Here, the nurse is leaving it in the arterial cannula.

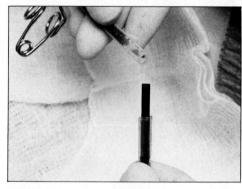

9 Now, insert a sterile adapter into the venous cannula.

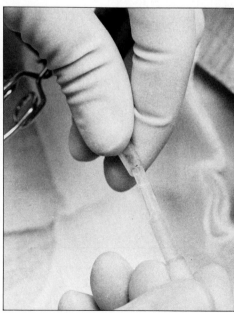

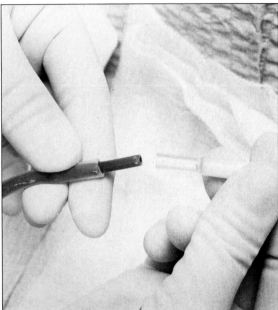

11 Next, insert the second shunt adapter over the Teflon connector in the arterial cannula.

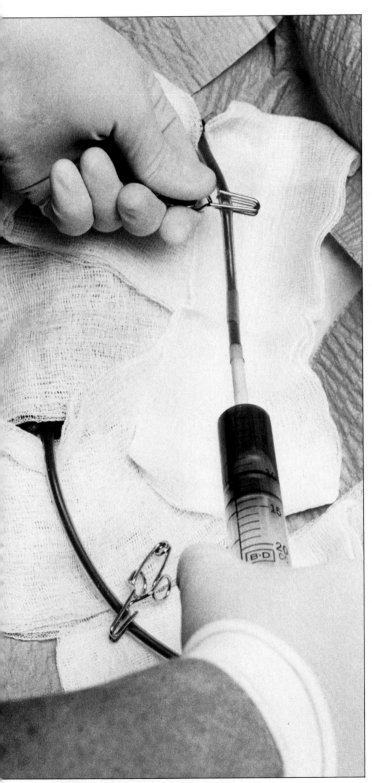

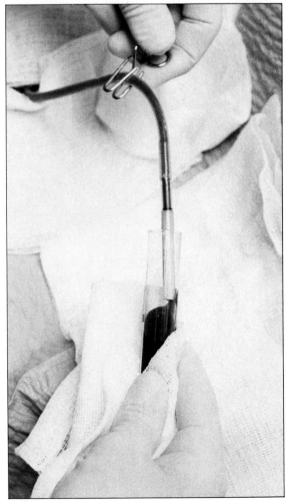

12 Withdraw a blood sample from the arterial cannula. If you need to use extra test tubes, have an assistant obtain them. But remember to hold them with a sterile gauze pad to avoid contaminating your sterile gloves. When you're finished, flush the cannula with the heparinized saline solution.

10 Attach the 20 cc syringe filled with heparinized saline solution to the venous cannula. Flush the cannula with the saline solution until the fluid in the cannula's almost clear.

Dialysis

Performing hemodialysis using an arteriovenous shunt continued

13 Now use a sterile gauze pad to grasp the arterial blood line on the dialysis machine. Attach the line to the arterial shunt adapter.

To start blood flowing, remove the bulldog clamp from the cannula. Have your assistant remove the tube-occluding clamp from the arterial line. She'll also check the dialysate temperature to make sure it's 98.6° F. (37° C.). If it is, she'll set the dialysate flow meter at 5 liters per minute. Then, she'll turn on the dialyzing machine, setting the blood flow rate at 90 to 120 ml per minute.

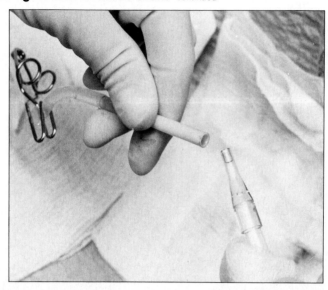

14 Now, before the blood flow reaches the venous blood line, connect the venous line to the venous shunt adapter. Then, remove the clamps on both the cannula and the blood line.

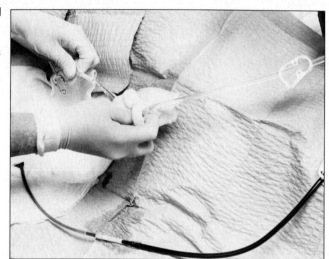

15 You may now remove your gloves. Tape the junction of the shunt adapter and the venous blood line so it's secure, leaving tabs on the ends of the tape. Also, tape the junction of the shunt adapter and cannula. Tape the arterial side of the shunt the same way.

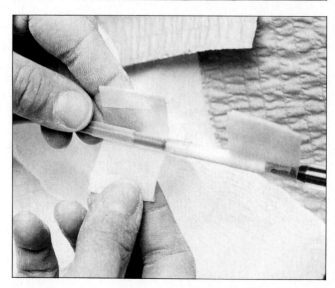

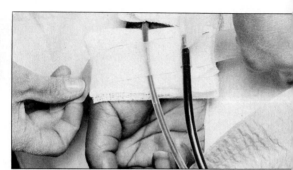

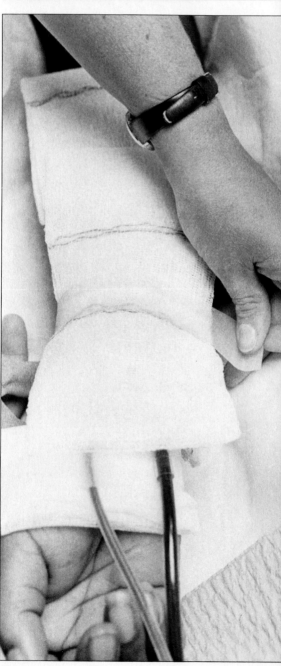

16 Remove the drape and gauze pads. Then, place three gauze pads lengthwise along the arm under the lines, overlapping them slightly. Fold a fourth pad and place under the lines nearest the patient's hand. Tape both lines securely, as shown here.

17 Put one unfolded gauze pad lengthwise over the others and tape it, as shown.

During hemodialysis, care for your patient following the guidelines on page 128.

When hemodialysis is completed, 3 to 6 hours later, disconnect the shunt from the hemodialysis machine, using aseptic technique. To do this, obtain sterile gloves, tube-occluding clamps, sterile bulldog clamps, povidone-iodine solution, sterile gauze pads, sterile alcohol swabs, tape, and an elastic bandage. Turn off the machine and reclamp the shunt cannulas. Put on your sterile gloves. Then, disconnect the machine blood lines.

Reconnect the shunt cannulas, taking care to position the Teflon shunt connector equally between the two cannulas. Otherwise, the cannula may become disconnected. Clean the shunt and its site with gauze pads soaked in povidone-iodine solution. Use alcohol swabs to clean off the povidone-iodine. Check the shunt to determine adequate blood flow. Apply a dressing to the shunt's site, and wrap it loosely with the elastic bandage.

After dialysis, weigh your patient and take her vital signs. Record this information on her dialysis record and in your nurses' notes. Also, record any lab studies for which you drew blood, and any special treatments given during dialysis, such as hypertonic mannitol infusion for muscle cramping. Also, record how the patient tolerated the entire procedure.

Nurses' guide to arteriovenous shunt complications

Complication	Signs and symptoms	Prevention	Treatment
Allergic reaction	• Rash, irritation, swelling, tenderness at exit sites	• Determine patient's allergy history before treatment begins.	• Discontinue use of irritant (usually antibiotic ointment).
Infection	• Redness, warmth, irritation, turgidity, tenderness, purulent drainage at exit sites • Pain at shunt site • Fever, or chills	• Perform daily care properly. • Observe aseptic technique when connecting and disconnecting shunt from hemodialysis machine.	• Inform doctor immediately. He'll order antibiotic therapy to prevent sepsis. • Observing aseptic technique, relieve symptoms with warm soaks. • If treatment is unsuccessful, the doctor must drain site and possibly move shunt.
Disconnected or separated shunts	• Blood leakage or severe hemorrhage	• Keep Teflon connector positioned exactly midway between the cannulas. • Keep shunt covered with dressings and elastic bandage. • Avoid bumping or knocking shunt. • Tell patient to avoid using arm with shunt too strenuously.	• In case of accidental separation of cannulas, apply bulldog clamps. Clean cannulas with povidone-iodine solution and carefully reconnect them with a new Teflon connector. • Suppose your patient's shunt cannulas have separate tip pieces. If separation occurs between the cannula and the tip, or the tip pulls out of the artery or vein, bulldog clamps won't work. Instead, apply a tourniquet or blood pressure cuff above the shunt site. Inflate the blood pressure cuff so that it applies pressure greater than the patient's systolic pressure. Call the doctor immediately.
Blood clotting	• Blood color change in shunt: bright red indicates normal flow; dark red to purple indicates beginning of clot formation; purplish red to black (with separation of purple cells and clear serum) indicates clotted shunt. • Weak bruit heard through stethoscope • Weak thrill on palpation • Blood temperature in shunt lower than normal	• Use only straight connectors, and avoid twisting or kinking tubing. • Monitor long shunts closely, since they're more likely to clot. • Take care to prevent infection, which can cause clotting. • Heparinize patient adequately. • Check for signs of fibrin formation (white specks in closed shunt, bloody threads in separated tubing. • If patient has hypotension, monitor him carefully. • Keep patient warm. • Observe patient carefully during hypercoagulable postoperative state.	• Inform the doctor immediately. He'll order anticoagulant therapy. • Gently aspirate shunt to remove blood clots. • Use a Fogarty embolectomy catheter to remove deep blood clots. *Note:* Only experienced personnel may use this equipment. • If treatment fails, doctor may revise shunt.

Dialysis

Performing hemodialysis using an arteriovenous fistula

1 *Grant Benson's a 60-year-old computer salesman who's been using a femoral catheter for hemodialysis while his fistula matures. Now that it has, you can insert fistula needles into it and attach them to a hemodialysis machine. One fistula needle will transport blood to the machine. The other will return dialyzed blood to the body. Read the following to find out how to perform the procedure.*

First, gather the following sterile equipment: two tube-occluding clamps, gloves, a 25G, ⅝" needle and a tuberculin syringe filled with lidocaine, ten 4"x4" gauze pads, two fistula needles with two attached 20 cc syringes filled with heparinized normal saline solution, two cotton-tipped applicators, and a test tube for a blood sample. Also, obtain povidone-iodine solution, nonallergenic tape, povidone-iodine ointment, a tourniquet, and a bed-saver pad (not shown).

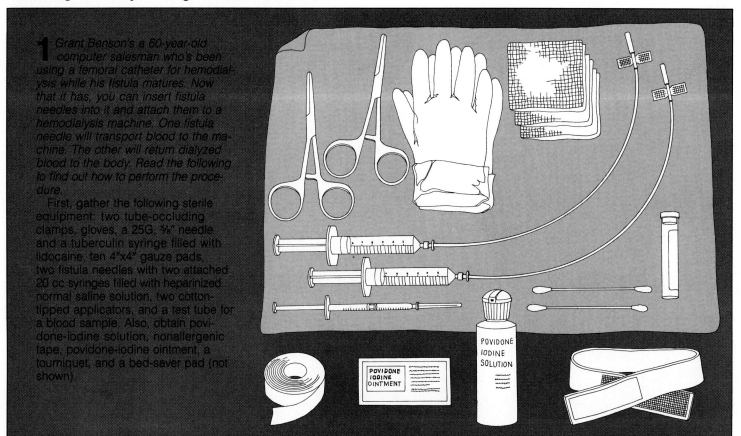

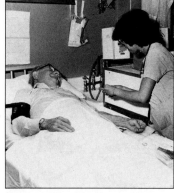

2 Explain the procedure to your patient. Then weigh him, and take his vital signs. Take his blood pressure while he's standing up and lying down. Record this information on the patient's dialysis record.

Make sure the machine is filled with dialysate and ready to turn on. Wash your hands.

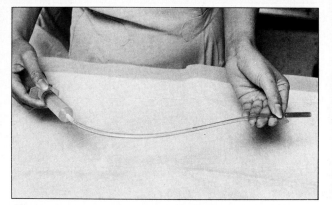

3 Prepare the fistula needles by flushing them with heparinized saline solution. Completely fill the tubing and needle to eliminate air bubbles.

Important: Leave the syringe attached to the fistula needle connector tubing and set this equipment aside. Don't allow it to become contaminated.

Note: If you need to draw blood for lab studies, don't use heparin in the first needle you insert, because the heparin could alter the lab results. Instead, insert a dry fistula needle. After insertion, draw the blood into a syringe. Use a tube-occluding clamp on the fistula needle tubing to control the blood flow. After you've drawn blood, attach a heparin-filled syringe and flush the needle and tubing.

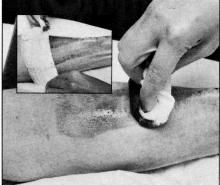

4 Now, you're ready to clean the fistula site. To begin, place a bed-saver pad under the patient's arm. Then, using a gauze pad soaked in povidone-iodine solution, make a 10" stroke down the arm over the fistula site. Use two more pads to make strokes on either side of the first stroke until you've cleaned a 3"-wide skin area.

[Inset] Then, use a dry gauze pad to dry off the povidone-iodine, as the nurse is doing here.

5 Now, apply a tourniquet to distend the veins for venipuncture. If the fistula's located in the wrist, place the tourniquet above the patient's elbow. But if the fistula's in the antecubital space, apply another tourniquet close to his shoulder.

Now, examine the blood vessels to find one that's full and resilient. Or, choose two vessels, one for the arterial needle and one for the venous needle.

Important: If your patient must undergo repeated hemodialysis treatments, vary venipuncture sites as much as possible.

7 Now you're ready to perform the venipuncture using the venous fistula needle. Remove the guard from one of the fistula needles. Then, squeeze the wing tips firmly together. Insert the venous needle at least 1″ above the fistula, in the direction of blood flow. As you do, angle the needle downward, but keep the bevel facing up. *Important:* Avoid puncturing the fistula.

Watch for blood backflow as the needle enters the blood vessel. Hold the syringe and plunger steady as you finish inserting the entire needle into the blood vessel.

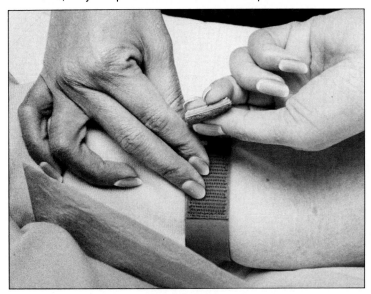

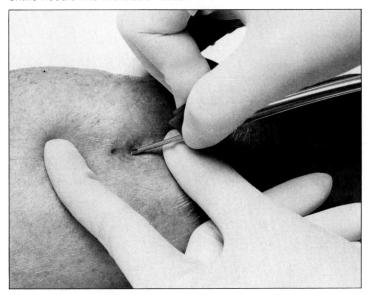

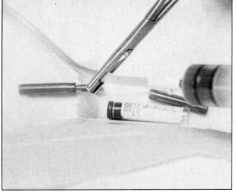

8 Now, release the tourniquet and, once again, flush the needle with heparinized saline solution to prevent clotting. Clamp the tubing with a tube-occluding clamp.

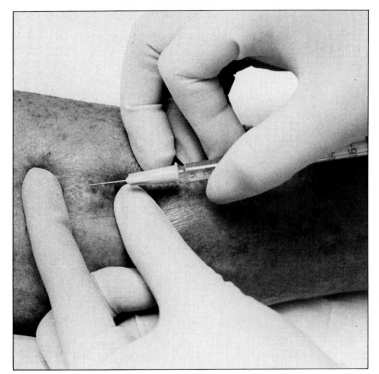

6 Put on sterile gloves. If the doctor orders, anesthetize the insertion site by injecting lidocaine just above the selected vein.

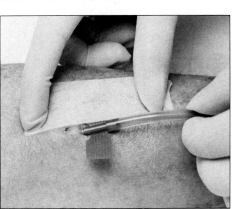

9 Use a 3″ length of nonallergenic tape to secure the needle, as shown.

Dialysis

Performing hemodialysis using an arteriovenous fistula continued

10 Apply a second 3″ length of tape to the needle site. Now you're ready to insert the arterial needle into the same blood vessel or another one you've chosen. To do this, repeat steps 6 through 10. However, this time insert the needle a few inches distal to the first needle, keeping the tip pointed away from the fistula.

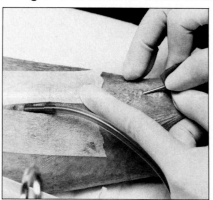

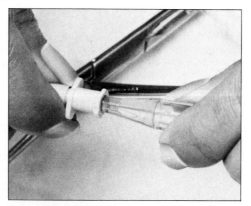

13 Now, attach the arterial needle tubing to the machine's arterial blood line. To do this, first remove the syringe from the end of the arterial needle tubing, then uncap the blood line tubing. Connect the arterial needle tubing to the blood line tubing.

11 Use cotton-tipped applicators to apply povidone-iodine ointment to the insertion sites.

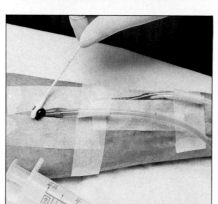

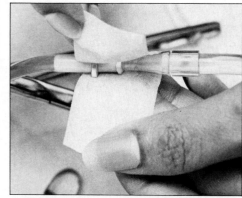

14 Tape the junction, as shown, leaving tabs at the end of the tape to ensure easy removal. To attach the venous needle tubing to the machine's venous blood line, repeat step 13 and tape the junction.

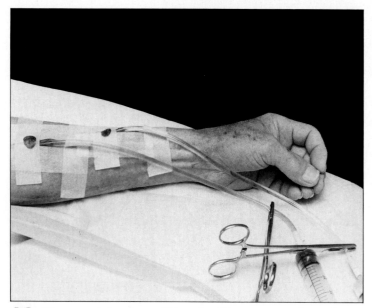

12 Then, apply two more 3″ lengths of tape over each needle insertion site, as shown.

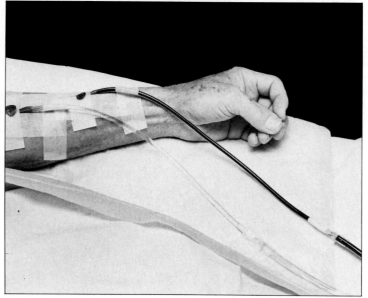

15 Before you begin the hemodialysis treatment, unclamp the venous and arterial needle tubings.
Now, check the temperature gauge on the machine to make sure the dialysate's at 98.6° F. (37° C.). Then, set the dialysate flow meter to 5 liters per minute. Remove the blood line clamps, and turn on the blood pump, setting it to pump 90 to 120 ml per minute.
Note the time you begin dialysis and document it. For patient care during dialysis, see page 128.

Discontinuing hemodialysis performed with an arteriovenous fistula

1 *Mr. Peter Johanessen, one of your end stage renal disease (ESRD) patients, has been undergoing hemodialysis for the past 4 hours. Now you must discontinue the treatment and remove the fistula needles. Here's how:*
First, gather the equipment shown in the inset: clean examining gloves, two adhesive bandage strips, two tube occluding clamps, and ten sterile 4"x4" gauze pads.
Remember to wash your hands.
Next, explain the procedure to your patient. Then, turn down the blood pump to 50 to 100 ml per minute. Put on the gloves.

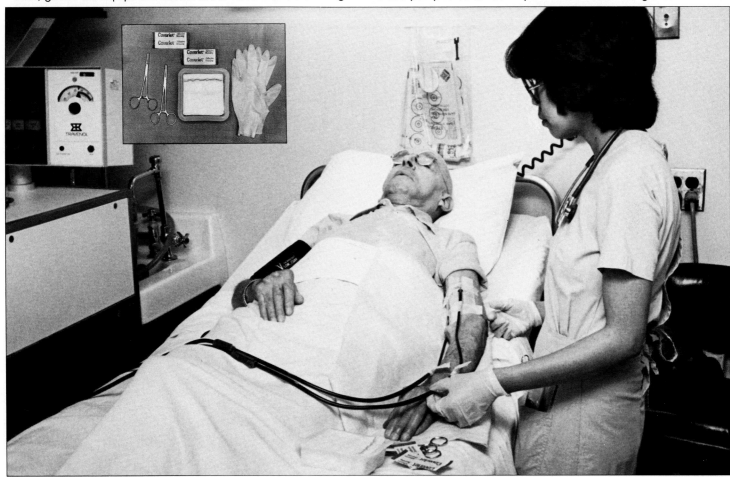

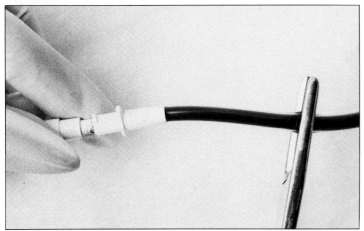

2 Remove the tape from the junction of the machine's arterial blood line and the needle tubing, and clamp the needle tubing.

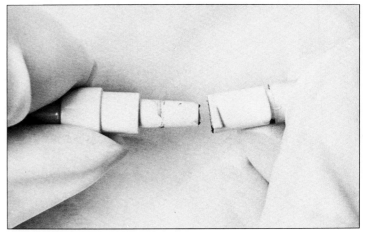

3 Disconnect the junction, as the nurse is doing here. The blood in the blood line will continue flowing toward the dialyzer, followed by a column of air.

Dialysis

Discontinuing hemodialysis performed with an arteriovenous fistula continued

4 Before the last of the blood reaches the T junction where the saline solution taps into the blood line, clamp the blood line. Quickly unclamp the saline solution line and allow solution to enter the line. Then, reclamp the saline solution line and unclamp the arterial line to allow a column of air to follow the blood and solution. The solution and air will help retransfuse the blood into the patient, so the minimum amount of blood remains in the equipment.

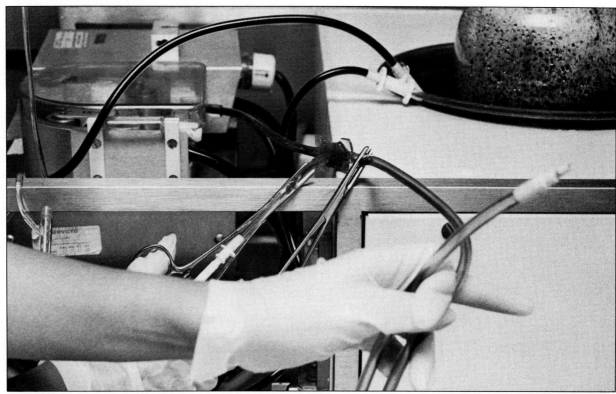

5 Allow blood to circulate through the system and reenter the patient's body through the venous needle tubing. But, before the last of the blood reenters the needle tubing, clamp the tubing.

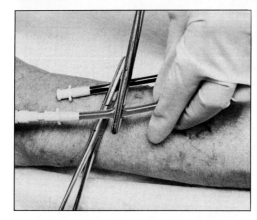

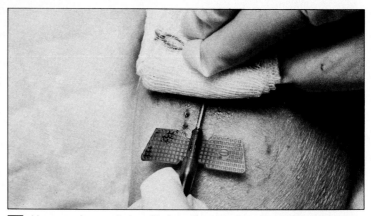

6 Then, clamp the machine's venous blood line, turn off the blood pump, and disconnect the line from the needle tubing.

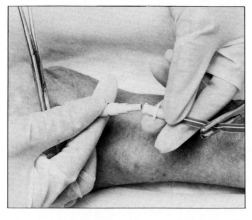

7 Now, you're ready to withdraw the needles. To do this, use one hand to hold a folded gauze pad over the venous venipuncture site. With your other hand, grasp the needle behind the wings and remove it. Immediately apply pressure to the site with the gauze pad for 3 to 5 minutes.

Note: If bleeding doesn't stop, apply direct pressure with a 7"x12" Upjohn Gelfoam® sterile sponge. If that doesn't help, apply a Gelfoam sponge soaked in topical thrombin solution.

When the bleeding stops, cover the site with an adhesive bandage strip. Repeat steps 6 and 7 for the arterial needle.

After hemodialysis, weigh your patient and take his vital signs. Record this information on his hemodialysis record and in your nurses' notes. Also, record any lab studies for which you drew blood, and any special treatments given during hemodialysis, such as hypertonic mannitol infusion for muscle cramping. Also, record how the patient tolerated the entire procedure.

Troubleshooting common arteriovenous (A-V) fistula problems

Although an arteriovenous (A-V) fistula causes fewer complications in hemodialysis patients than an A-V shunt, problems do arise. Vascular inadequacy, poor surgical technique, or reduced blood volume may cause primary fistula failure. Secondary fistula failure may develop from blood clotting, tissue infiltration, or aneurysm. If the fistula fails for any reason, the doctor may have to alter the fistula (fistula revision), create a new fistula, or implant a vein graft. If these measures don't work, as a last resort, he may have to insert a shunt.

Even if a fistula functions well at first, infection may occur at the venipuncture sites. An infection may lead to blood clotting, septicemia, or subacute bacterial endocarditis (SBE).

Also, some patients develop fistula *steal syndrome.* This syndrome occurs when an inadequate supply of blood reaches the hand because the fistula has redirected the arterial supply. Warm, moist compresses or physical therapy may relieve minor symptoms, but severe steal syndrome can cause gangrene. To prevent this outcome in severe cases, the doctor may revise the fistula.

Problem	Possible causes	Nursing action
Sluggish blood flow	• Needle bevel against wall of blood vessel	• Pull needle back slightly to alter bevel's position. • Or, place gauze pad under needle hub to lift bevel away from vessel wall. • Or, rotate needle so bevel points downward.
	• Needle too large for blood vessel	• Replace needle with one of correct size (higher gauge number).
	• Low vascular pressure	• Reapply tourniquet temporarily.
	• Needle out of alignment	• Realign needle correctly.
	• Clotted needle	• Replace needle.
Needle tubing collapse	• Vasospasm	• Realign needle. • Decrease blood flow rate slightly. If spasm occurs during every hemodialysis treatment, patient should soak arm or leg with fistula in warm water for 10 to 15 minutes before hemodialysis. • The doctor may order a vasodilator such as nylidrin hydrochloride (Arlidin*), to relieve vasospasm.
	• Needle out of alignment	• Realign needle correctly.
Needle slipping out of blood vessel	• Improper taping	• Turn off blood pump. Clamp both arterial and venous lines and apply pressure over venipuncture site until bleeding stops (about 5 to 15 minutes). • Reinsert new needle into blood vessel and tape securely.
Hematoma formation	• Needle has punctured both walls of blood vessel.	• After hemodialysis, remove needle. Then use a sterile gauze pad to stop bleeding. Apply cool, moist compresses until heparin effects wear off (4 to 6 hours after hemodialysis). Then, apply warm, moist compresses to relieve soreness and help reabsorption of the hematoma.
Excessive bleeding	• Needle too large	• Replace needle with one of correct size.
	• Needle has punctured both walls of blood vessel; or repeated puncture of thin, dry skin	• Apply direct pressure for 3 to 5 minutes immediately after hemodialysis. Use Gelfoam sponges if bleeding persists. The doctor may also order protamine sulfate to counteract heparin. If so, inject the sulfate slowly.
	• Excessive use of heparin	• Reduce heparin dosage.

*Available in both the United States and in Canada

Dialysis

Caring for a patient during hemodialysis

• Immediately after you begin hemodialysis at the blood flow rate of 90 to 120 ml per minute, check the patient's blood pressure and vital signs. If these are stable, increase the pump speed to 150 ml per minute. Then, if you're using minimal or intermittent heparinization, inject the heparin loading dose into the injection port on the arterial blood line. The loading dose will range from 1,000 to 3,000 units, depending on the equipment used.

  However, if the blood pressure is unstable, don't increase the blood flow rate beyond 90 ml per minute. Also, reduce the ultrafiltration pressure by turning down the negative-pressure dial on the negative-pressure machine, or by loosening the clamp on the venous blood line on a positive-pressure machine.
• No matter what your patient's blood pressure is, check it again in 5 minutes. If it remains stable, increase the blood flow rate by 50 to 100 ml per minute. If your patient with unstable blood pressure has now stabilized, inject the heparin loading dose and proceed as usual.Repeat the blood pressure checks and the blood flow rate increases until you reach the desired flow rate of 300 ml per minute. Maintain this flow rate throughout hemodialysis.
• After the maintenance blood flow rate has been achieved, you're ready to adjust the ultrafiltration pressure. If you're using a negative-pressure machine, calculate the desired fluid loss by subtracting the patient's ideal weight from his current weight. Set the ultrafiltration pressure accordingly.
• If you're using a coil dialyzer (pictured to the right) with a positive-pressure machine, check the patient's weight record to find out the fluid loss at his last dialysis. Note the pressure setting used. Compare the weight lost during his last dialysis with his ideal weight. If the fluid loss was insufficient, increase the positive pressure to a level as high as his blood pressure will permit without causing hypovolemia and hypotension. Do so by tightening the Hoffman clamp on the venous blood line. Then, read the venous pressure gauge to determine the resulting ultrafiltration pressure increase.
• If you're using a hollow fiber artificial kidney (HFAK) dialyzer, turn it upside down. This position helps the blood move through the semipermeable membrane, particularly during retransfusion.

• At least once every half hour, record the patient's vital signs (more frequently if his condition changes).
• Once each hour, check the patient's blood pressure and check the arterial and venous pressure gauges. Record negative pressure, and reduce it if the patient's hypotensive.
• Once each hour, check the patient's blood clotting time by drawing a blood sample and obtaining a Lee-White-method clotting time. Inject heparin into the system as the clotting times dictate.
• Also, periodically check the blood lines for clotting. If the lines are clotted, check your patient's dialysis record to find his clotting time. If you haven't obtained a clotting time within the past half hour, obtain one. Inject heparin as the clotting time indicates.
• Periodically check blood lines to make sure junctions are secure.
• Check patient's hydration level and infuse or remove fluid as needed.

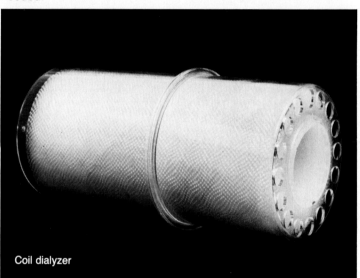

Coil dialyzer

Learning about diet for the hemodialysis patient

The diet of a hemodialysis patient critically affects his condition and progress. Because the metabolic rate of a patient with renal failure slows down, he must alter his eating habits significantly. For example:
• He must limit his protein intake because protein breaks down into toxic nitrogen waste that's difficult for an impaired kidney to filter out of the blood. But, because protein's essential for body tissue growth and replacement, too little will also be detrimental. Depending on the patient's creatinine clearance level, the doctor will probably put him on a diet that initially limits his protein intake to about 40 to 60 grams daily. After hemodialysis treatments start, daily protein intake may be increased to about 60 to 80 grams, equivalent to that of a normal, adequately nourished individual.
• He must limit his sodium intake because it causes water retention, which leads to hypertension. A hemodialysis patient should ingest no more than 2 grams sodium per day. This limit should keep his blood pressure stable throughout the hemodialysis program.
• He must limit his potassium intake because his impaired kidneys can't eliminate enough potassium. Too much potassium affects myocardial function adversely. But, because a certain amount of potassium is necessary, too little can also cause problems. Keep the

patient's potassium intake from 1.5 to 2 grams daily so that his serum potassium level doesn't fall below 3.5 mEq/liter.

  Of course, no diet would be well planned without considering caloric and fluid intake. Usually the renal failure patient will be underweight, because his illness has impaired his appetite. Also, because his protein intake is restricted, he'll have to increase his caloric intake to prevent his body from using what little protein he ingests (or from drawing on muscle tissue) for energy.

  For a time, his weight may remain constant from fluid retention. But that's only temporary. A proper diet is needed to replace fluid weight with solid weight. Make sure your patient takes in 3,000 calories a day, roughly 700 calories more than a normal daily intake for a well-nourished person. Decrease his caloric intake, if needed, as he gains weight.

  Also, restrict his fluid intake to 500 to 1,000 ml per day, so fluid retention doesn't become a problem.

  After the hospital dietitian, working with the doctor, develops a proper diet for your patient, discuss it with him. If your hospital or dialysis-equipment manufacturer supplies a diet booklet, give a copy to your patient. This will help him understand the importance of diet and will provide answers to his questions.

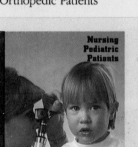
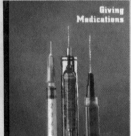
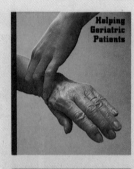
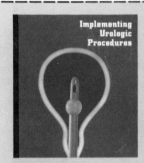
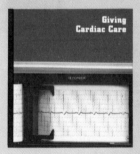
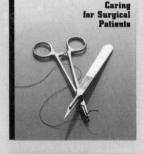
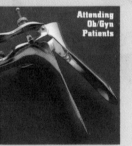
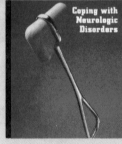
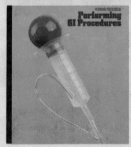
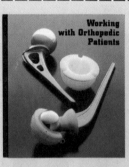
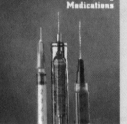

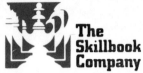
Introduce yourself to the popular NURSING PHOTOBOOK™ series

Each book in this unique series contains detailed *photostories*…and diagrams, charts, and anatomic illustrations to help you learn important new procedures. And each handsome PHOTOBOOK offers you • 160 illustrated, fact-filled pages • clear, close-up photographs • convenient 9″ × 10½″ size • durable, hardcover binding • complete index. Watch the experts at work showing you how to… administer drugs…teach your patient about his illness and its treatment…minimize trauma… increase patient comfort…and more. Discover how you can become a better nurse by joining this exciting series. You can examine each PHOTOBOOK at your leisure… for 10 days *absolutely free*! Even if you've paid and later decide a PHOTOBOOK is not really helpful, you can return it at any time in the next 2 years, and we'll refund your money.

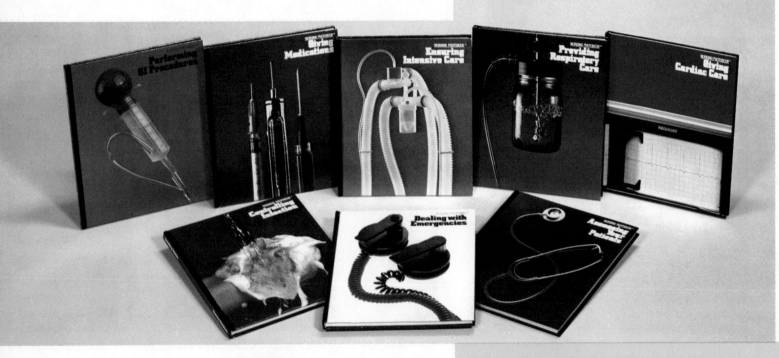

At last! A magazine that helps you with "the other side" of nursing. The things they didn't (and couldn't) teach you in nursing school.

NursingLife tells you how to be a better nurse…how to find greater fulfillment in your career…how to grow on the job.

It's about the *nonclinical* skills today's nurses need to round out their professional lives.

Become a Charter Subscriber to this exciting new magazine. Just tear off and mail this card today. There's no need to send money now. This is a no-obligation, free-trial offer!

If order card is missing, send your order to:

NursingLife®

P.O. Box 1961
One Health Care Circle
Marion, Ohio 43305

Learning about medications for the hemodialysis patient

As you know, the kidneys play a major role in metabolizing and excreting medication. That's why you must take care administering medication to a patient with renal failure.

If the renal failure patient's on hemodialysis, he'll probably be receiving:

• Aluminum hydroxide, to control his phosphorus level (by binding with phosphates in his gastrointestinal tract). However, never give an aluminum hydroxide preparation containing magnesium, for example, Gelusil®, or the magnesium will accumulate and cause magnesium toxicosis.

• Calcium supplements, to compensate for calcium deficiency.

• Iron preparations, to combat iron depletion. *Caution:* Never administer iron and aluminum hydroxide at the same time, because aluminum hydroxide hinders iron absorption. Instead, give the iron preparation earlier or later.

• Multivitamins and folic-acid tablets to supplement his diet. Don't administer the multivitamin capsules immediately before hemodialysis because the vitamins will be eliminated during the procedure.

Your patient may be taking additional drugs for other complications associated with renal failure; for example, for infection, heart disease, and mental depression. In most cases, the doctor will prescribe far less than average doses for these conditions because of the patient's slowed metabolic rate.

Slowed metabolic rate and reduced clearance through the kidneys are the main reasons why the renal failure patient will have more medication side effects than other patients. Stay alert for such problems and notify the doctor if they occur.

Tell the patient the name and dose for each prescribed drug and explain the drug's purpose and possible side effects. If the patient's going home, emphasize the importance of taking his medications on schedule. Warn him not to take any medications, including those sold over the counter, without contacting his doctor.

Nurses' guide to hemodialysis complications

COMPLICATIONS	POSSIBLE CAUSES	NURSING CONSIDERATIONS
Internal hemorrhage	• Excessive heparinization	• Decrease initial heparin dose; or use minimal or regional heparinization. • Observe patient for signs of internal bleeding: apprehension; restlessness; pale, cold, clammy skin; excessive thirst; decreased blood pressure; rapid, weak, and thready pulse; increased respirations; decreased temperature. • Doctor may order blood transfusions.
External hemorrhage	• Line disconnection	• Observe blood lines for leakage. • Keep clamps ready in case any line disconnects. • Keep blood pressure cuff nearby to use as a tourniquet.
Aggravated anemia	• Blood loss in hemodialyzer lines and equipment	• Doctor may order blood transfusions, folic acid, and iron.
Hepatitis	• Blood transfusion with infected blood	• Take care not to infect patient when performing blood transfusions and dialysis: wear gloves, particularly if you have an open wound; cap all needles; observe strict aseptic technique. • If patient has hepatitis, keep him in isolation during hemodialysis. • Patient should be tested every 4 weeks for hepatitis; staff should be tested every 3 months.
Dialysis disequilibrium syndrome (headache, fatigue, muscle agitation, twitching, and confusion, possibly leading to grand mal seizure)	• Rapid shift of fluid and electrolyte levels	• Slow blood flow rate during hemodialysis. • Inform doctor immediately; he may order diazepam (Valium*), or phenytoin sodium (Dilantin*), or discontinue therapy. • Doctor may order other treatment, such as analgesics, for symptoms.
Hypotension	• Septic shock • Reduced blood volume from extracorporeal circulation • Poor cardiac output	• Place the patient in Trendelenburg's position. • Infuse normal saline solution, as necessary, to restore blood volume. • Doctor may order mannitol infusion. • Doctor may order plasma or albumin infusion. • Check blood pressure every 10 minutes until it stabilizes.
Cardiac arrhythmia or angina	• Rapid shift of fluid and electrolyte levels • Reduced blood volume, from extracorporeal circulation • Reduced hematocrit level	• If hyperkalemia is the cause, doctor will order sodium polystyrene sulfonate (Kayexalate*). • If decreased blood volume is the cause, the doctor will order blood transfusions. • Doctor may order antiarrhythmics, for example, lidocaine (Xylocaine*), or procainamide hydrochloride (Pronestyl*).
Muscle cramping	• Rapid shift of fluid and electrolyte levels	• Doctor may order normal saline solution infused with 100 ml 25% mannitol, 10 ml 23% sodium chloride, or 50 ml 50% dextrose.
Lower back pain	• Blood flow rate too rapid at start of hemodialysis	• Reduce initial blood flow rate. • Doctor may order diphenhydramine hydrochloride (Benadryl*).
Air embolism	• Insufficient blood flow • I.V. bag empty • Loose connections	• Monitor blood flow rate carefully. • Hang bags rather than bottles of dialysate, because bags are less likely to admit air into tubing. • Clamp I.V. line before bag empties. • Make sure tubing connections are secure. • If patient's blood pressure falls rapidly, if he has a weak, rapid pulse, and he is cyanotic, turn him on his left side and lower the head of the bed. This position will help keep on the right side of his heart any air that's entered, so that the pulmonary artery can absorb air bubbles. Notify the doctor immediately.

*Available in both the United States and in Canada

Dialysis

Performing peritoneal dialysis with a temporary catheter: Initial steps

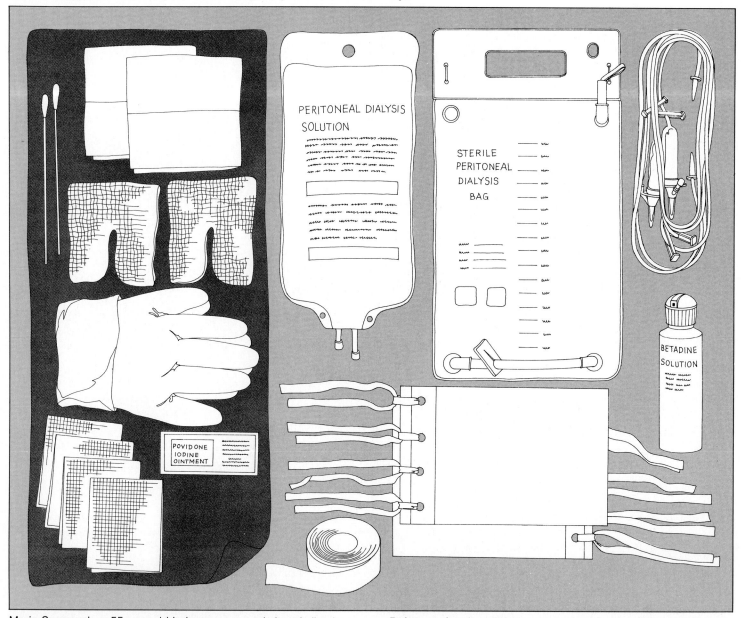

Maria Spanacek, a 55-year-old baker, was recently hospitalized with circulatory collapse. Acute renal failure quickly set in as a secondary complication. Because her cardiovascular condition contraindicates hemodialysis, the doctor has inserted a temporary catheter for performing peritoneal dialysis.

To perform peritoneal dialysis, first assemble the sterile equipment shown here: two cotton-tipped applicators, two precut Surgipads, four 4"x4" gauze pads, two precut 4"x4" gauze pads, gloves, and povidone-iodine ointment. Also, gather the nonsterile equipment shown: 2-liter bag of peritoneal dialysate, 3-way tubing, povidone-iodine (Betadine) solution, nonallergenic tape, Montgomery straps, and a dialysis drainage bag. Obtain an I.V. pole (not shown).

Remember to wash your hands.

Explain the procedure to your patient. Weigh her, and take her vital signs, including her blood pressure while she's standing up and lying down. Record this information on her dialysis record.

Before performing dialysis, you must spike the dialysate bag with the tubing.

Note: If the doctor's ordered any medication, inject it into the injection port on the bag before spiking the bag.

Then, close all clamps on the tubing. Pull off the protective cover from the bag's outflow port and insert the spike into the port.

Now, you'll prime the tubing to eliminate possible air bubbles. Do so by opening the clamp near the dialysate bag. Also, open the clamp on the short piece of tubing beyond the Y. (You'll connect this piece to the patient's catheter during the procedure.) Make sure the clamp on the longer half of the Y (which you'll connect to the drainage bag) stays closed. Also, keep the unused spike tubing clamp closed.

Allow the dialysate to flow from the end of the short tubing. Then, close the clamps.

Finally, hang the bag on the I.V. pole.

Performing peritoneal dialysis with a temporary catheter: The procedure

1 *After you've gathered the equipment and primed the tubing, you're ready to begin preparing the catheter for dialysis.*

First, remove the dressing from the patient's abdomen. Check the catheter insertion site for redness, swelling, or other signs of infection or irritation.

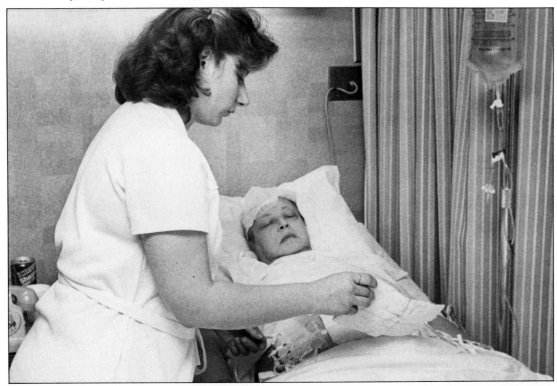

2 Now, you're ready to clean the catheter site. To do so, pour povidone-iodine solution over three sterile 4"x4" gauze pads. Then, put on sterile gloves. Using a soaked gauze pad, begin cleaning the skin around the catheter insertion site. Move outward from the base of the catheter insertion site in a circular motion. Complete the cleaning with a second gauze pad, until you've cleaned a 2" radius around the insertion site.

3 Next, use a gauze pad soaked in povidone-iodine solution to clean the catheter itself, moving in one direction only, from the insertion site to the end of the catheter.

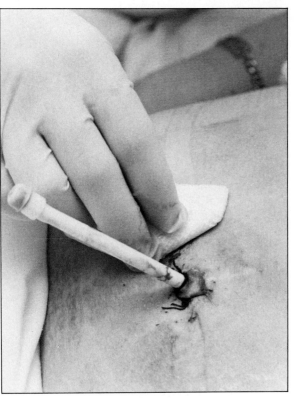

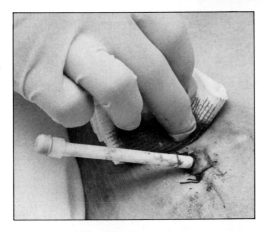

4 After you've finished cleaning the catheter, use a new sterile gauze pad to gently pat dry the skin and the catheter.

Dialysis

Performing peritoneal dialysis with a temporary catheter: The procedure continued

5 When the skin and catheter are completely dry, use a cotton-tipped applicator to apply povidone-iodine ointment to the insertion site.

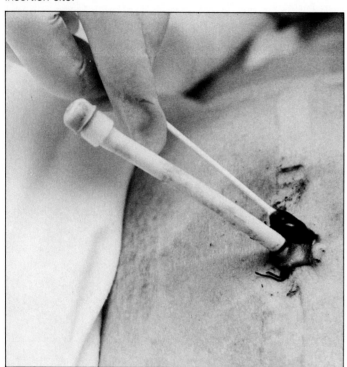

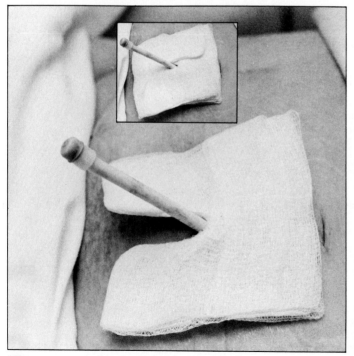

6 Now, you're ready to apply the dressing. First, lay down a precut gauze pad around the catheter.
[Inset] Then, lay down a second precut gauze pad so that it's facing the opposite direction.

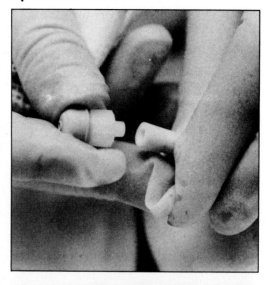

7 Next, you'll connect the catheter to the dialysate tubing. To do so, remove the catheter cap.

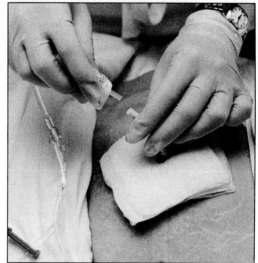

8 Now, pick up the dialysate tubing, using a gauze pad. Remove the cap from the tubing. Now, connect the catheter to the tubing.

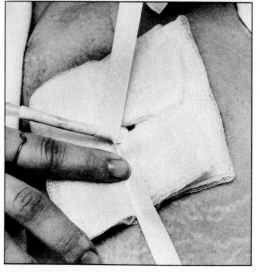

9 Remove gloves. Then, wind two 12″ lengths of tape around the tubing to secure it to the abdomen, as shown here.

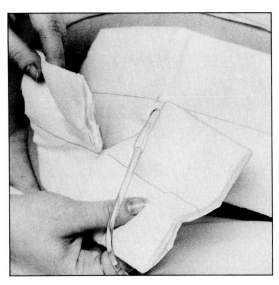

10 Now, apply the two precut Surgipads, laying them down so each one faces the opposite direction.

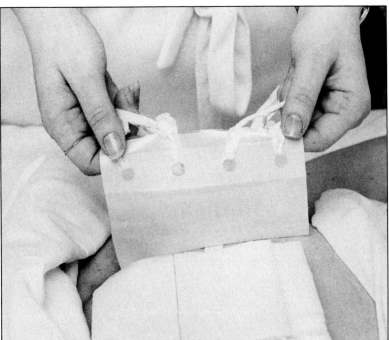

11 Cover the dressing with Montgomery straps and secure the strings. Then, open the two clamps that control dialysate flow into the patient. Allow the dialysate 5 to 10 minutes to drain into the peritoneum. Just before all the dialysate's drained into the peritoneum, close both clamps on the dialysate inflow tubing. Doing this will keep air from entering the line.

The dialysate may remain in the patient's peritoneum for approximately 1½ hours. When this time is up, open the clamp to the drainage bag. Allow 10 to 20 minutes for the dialysate to drain out. Then, close the clamp.

Now, obtain a new bag of dialysate. Remove the spike from the empty bag and insert it in the new bag. Hang the new bag on the I.V. pole. Then, begin a new exchange cycle by opening the two clamps that control dialysate flow into the patient's abdomen. Perform the number of exchanges the doctor has ordered.

Performing patient care during peritoneal dialysis treatment

To care for a patient receiving peritoneal dialysis treatment, follow these guidelines:
• At the beginning of the procedure, monitor his vital signs every 10 minutes until they stabilize. Then, since pressure from fluid in his abdomen can affect blood pressure, check the patient's vital signs each time dialysate drains.

Note: Warm solution in the abdomen may increase body temperature.
• Obtain cultures of dialysis drainage after the first and last exchange; or after 8- to 12-hour intervals during a long treatment; or if you see signs of infection.
• Following the therapeutic goal established for your patient, determine the amount of fluid that should be removed during each exchange and the balance required at the end of each treatment. Maintain records to determine if the patient is in positive balance (retaining some infused dialysate) or negative balance (more fluid returned than infused) for each exchange.
• Care for the patient's skin and change his position frequently. Provide passive range of motion exercises and encourage deep breathing and coughing. This care will give comfort, decrease chance of tissue breakdown, and enhance dialysate drainage.
• Provide adequate nutrition, following the prescribed diet (if your patient has one). Remember, your patient's condition is catabolic, and he is debilitated. Protein losses across the peritoneal membrane are great, so the patient requires replacement protein for tissue repair and maintenance.
• Calculate the patient's total fluid balance at the end of each treatment, or after 8-hour intervals during a long treatment. Include both oral and I.V. fluid intake, as well as urinary output. Estimate or calculate any other fluid output, such as wound drainage or perspiration.

Disconnecting a temporary catheter

After you've performed the prescribed number of exchanges, you must disconnect your patient's catheter from the peritoneal dialysis system. Assemble sterile gloves, a sterile 4"x4" gauze pad, a sterile protective (injection) cap, sterile Surgipads, nonallergenic tape, and Montgomery straps.
• Open the sterile equipment. Then, put on the gloves. With one hand, pick up the sterile gauze pad and grasp the end of the tubing with it.
• With your other hand, grasp the catheter. Now, gently disconnect the tubing from the catheter.
• Next, put the protective cap on the catheter.
• Place an uncut Surgipad over the catheter. Tape it in place, and cover the dressing with Montgomery straps.
• Weigh your patient and take his vital signs. Also, calculate his total fluid balance, as indicated earlier on this page. Record this information on his peritoneal dialysis record and in your nurses' notes.

Dialysis

Learning about the Tenckhoff catheter

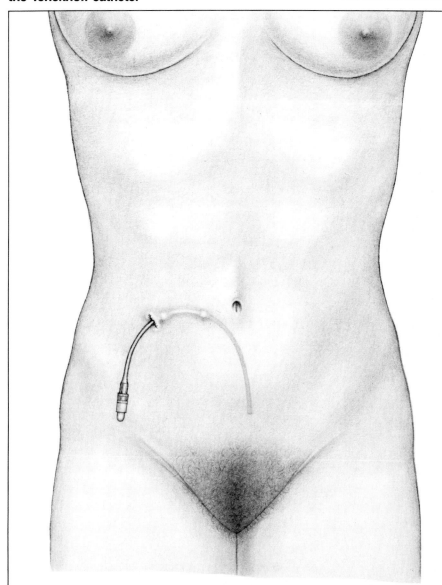

Maria Spanacek, your acute renal failure patient, had a temporary cathether inserted for peritoneal dialysis. But, an end stage renal disease (ESRD) patient using peritoneal dialysis will have a permanent (Tenckhoff) catheter surgically implanted. This catheter, pictured above, significantly reduces the risk of peritonitis.

To implant this 34 cm catheter, the doctor inserts the first 17 cm of it into the patient's abdomen. The next 7 cm segment, which the doctor tunnels subcutaneously, has a Dacron cuff at each end. Within a few days after insertion, the patient's tissues grow closely around these Dacron cuffs, forming a tight barrier against bacterial invasion. The remaining 10 cm of the catheter extends outside the abdomen. The external tip of the catheter is equipped with a metal adapter so it can be connected to dialysate tubing.

The patient with a Tenckhoff catheter can use any of three dialysis systems: a dialysate bag, tubing, and drainage-bag set, as for the temporary catheter; a continuous ambulatory peritoneal dialysis (CAPD) bag-and-tubing set (see the following pages); or, a dialysate delivery machine, which automatically administers dialysate exchanges.

Learning about continuous ambulatory peritoneal dialysis

If your end stage renal disease (ESRD) patient is highly motivated and responsible, he probably can use continuous ambulatory peritoneal dialysis (CAPD). In this form of dialysis, the dialysate remains in the patient's peritoneum 24 hours a day, 7 days a week. As the procedure's name indicates, the patient can be ambulatory throughout treatment; he's not confined to a bed or connected to a machine.

Although the risk of peritonitis is great with CAPD, this procedure maintains serum chemistries, electrolytes, and hematocrit within acceptable limits. It rarely creates serious blood pressure problems and doesn't require expensive equipment. The patient himself can perform almost all the necessary procedures, and can usually learn them within 2 weeks. Because the patient can move about freely during treatment, this dialysis method disrupts his lifestyle very little. All these advantages contribute to the increasing use of CAPD by end stage renal disease patients.

The CAPD method involves the peritoneal cavity, a permanently implanted Tenckhoff catheter, connecting tubing, and a collapsible dialysate bag.

After the doctor inserts the Tenckhoff catheter, 48-hour peritoneal dialysis treatment with 1,000 ml hourly exchanges is immediately initiated. An exchange entails draining used dialysate from the abdomen and instilling fresh dialysate. Between exchanges dialysate remains in the abdomen.

On the third day after insertion, the patient begins a regimen of five exchanges a day for 1 week, using dialysate with 1.5% dextrose concentration and added antibiotics, usually cephalothin sodium (Keflin Neutral*) and tobramycin sulfate (Nebcin*). Heparin and lidocaine may also be added.

In the second week, the daily exchanges decrease to three. The patient uses dialysate with a 1.5% dextrose concentration for the first two exchanges, and dialysate with a 4.25% dextrose concentration for the third exchange if his weight gain indicates he's retaining too much fluid. During the day, these exchanges last from 6 to 8 hours. The night exchange lasts from 8 to 12 hours, so the patient can sleep without interruption. The doctor may prescribe a fourth or fifth exchange.

You may begin training the patient to perform his own peritoneal dialysis exchanges toward the end of his first week of peritoneal dialysis. Your instruction should include mechanics of peritoneal dialysis, aseptic technique, performing a dialysis exchange, daily catheter care, complications, diet, medications, monitoring weight and vital signs, ordering supplies, and record keeping.

Give your patient a copy of the sample daily record on page 141. His copy will show him how to fill out the form he'll use during the first 2 months of his CAPD program. After that, he'll use a weekly record form.

The patient on peritoneal dialysis requires almost no medication, and has few diet restrictions. But, the doctor will prescribe multiple vitamins and a folic-acid supplement, to replace losses across the peritoneal membrane. Also, because the peritoneal dialysis patient loses much more protein across the peritoneal membrane than the hemodialysis patient loses across the dialyzer, the peritoneal dialysis patient must ingest more protein than the ESRD patient. Each day, he should consume 1 gram of protein per kilogram of body weight. In addition, the patient should increase his potassium intake (to replace losses), and reduce his sodium intake (if he retains fluid).

CAPD's primary disadvantage is the increased risk of peritonitis, which can lead to septic shock and death. In addition, a number of minor complications, such as asymptomatic hernia and lower back pain, may occur. To help prevent peritonitis, you must teach your patient aseptic technique. Specifically, he must learn how to perform a dialysate exchange (which involves draining used dialysate and transferring the tubing spike to a new bag of dialysate) without contaminating the spike. To help teach your patient proper technique, use the home care aid on pages 138 to 140.

If a patient develops signs and symptoms of peritonitis, he probably can be treated as an outpatient. First, he'll collect his own drainage samples for culture and cell count. If the culture and cell count confirm the infection, the doctor will order antibiotic therapy. He'll order hospitalization if the patient doesn't improve within 24 to 36 hours, or if the patient can't perform dialysis because the dialysate won't drain in or out. (See the chart on pages 142 to 143 for information on peritonitis and other complications of peritoneal dialysis.)

Performing a tubing change for a continuous ambulatory peritoneal dialysis patient

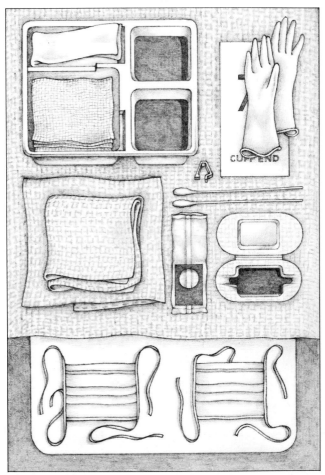

1 *Continuous ambulatory peritoneal dialysis (CAPD) patients can perform most necessary procedures themselves. But once a month your CAPD patient will require a change of tubing. The following photostory tells you how to perform this procedure.*

Begin by assembling the sterile equipment shown here: peritoneal catheter clamp, Clinitub™ filled with povidone-iodine solution, pediatric urine collector, and a peritoneal dialysis on-off tray, including povidone-iodine solution, two 300 ml prep cups, gloves, two cotton-tipped applicators, 10 4"x4" gauze pads, and three drapes. Also obtain this equipment: tubing, a 2-liter bag of peritoneal dialysate, two masks, and an I.V. pole.

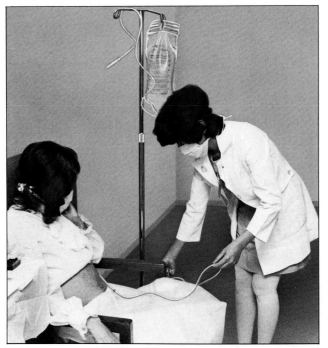

2 Explain the procedure to your patient. Record her vital signs, including her blood pressure while she's standing up and lying down. Then, seat her comfortably in a chair. Lay a bed-saver pad on her lap. Put masks on her and yourself.

Remember to wash your hands thoroughly with povidone-iodine scrub solution.

Dialysis

Performing a tubing change for a continuous ambulatory peritoneal dialysis patient continued

3 Spike the dialysate bag with the new tubing. Hang the bag on an I.V. pole and prime the tubing by opening the roller clamp. Uncap the tubing and allow the dialysate to flow through the tubing to eliminate possible air bubbles. Tape the capped tubing to the I.V. pole to keep the tubing out of your way.

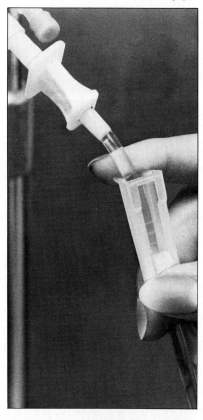

4 Next, have the patient remove the empty bag from her clothing and position it below her abdomen to drain out the used dialysate. While she's doing this, open your sterile equipment and put on the sterile gloves. So you don't contaminate your gloves, use a sterile gauze pad to pick up the tubing as you place a sterile drape, shiny, coated side down, on the patient's lap.

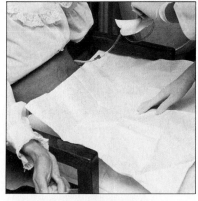

5 Now, you're ready to clean the catheter exit site. First, soak the gauze pads with povidone-iodine solution. Holding the catheter with a *dry* gauze pad, use a *soaked* pad to clean in a circular motion from the exit site outward. Continue the cleaning with two more gauze pads, using a different pad for each stroke, until you've cleaned in a 2″ radius.

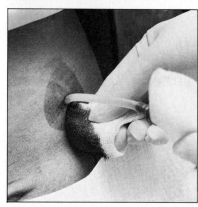

6 Use another povidone-iodine-soaked gauze pad to clean the catheter, moving in one direction only, from the exit site to the catheter-tubing junction. To complete the cleaning, repeat this step with a second gauze pad.

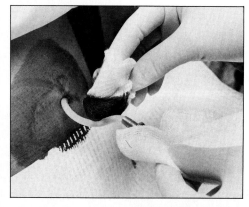

7 Then, use a dry gauze pad to blot excess povidone-iodine from the catheter and skin. Finish blotting with a second gauze pad until all of the povidone-iodine solution is absorbed.

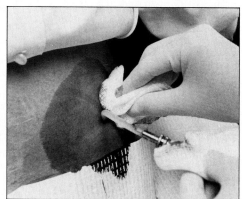

8 Now, set the Clinitub on the sterile drape on the patient's lap. Place the catheter-tubing junction in the tub and close the lid. Be sure to submerge the junction completely, or rotate the junction several times while soaking it.

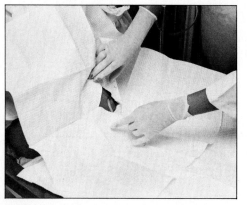

9 After 5 minutes, remove the catheter-tubing junction from the tub. Let the junction rest on the sterile drape as you fill up a pediatric urine collector with povidone-iodine solution. Position a precut drape over the catheter exit site, as shown here.

10 Now, clamp the catheter 1″ proximal to the junction.

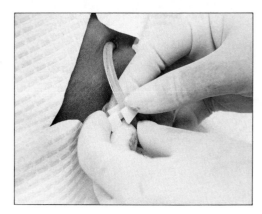

11 Disconnect the catheter from the tubing. Temporarily cover the end of the catheter with a gauze pad to prevent contamination while you peel the tape from the adhesive faceplate of the pediatric urine collector.

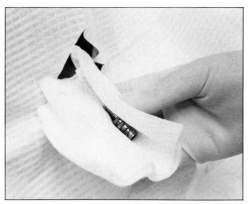

12 Remove the gauze pad and insert the end of the catheter into the povidone-iodine-filled pediatric urine collector. Apply the adhesive faceplate to the patient's abdomen.

After 10 minutes, remove the pediatric urine collector.

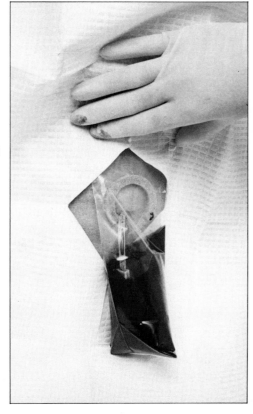

13 Now, wrap another gauze pad around the catheter. Place a third drape on the patient's lap, under the catheter.

Use a cotton-tipped applicator to dry the metal catheter tip.

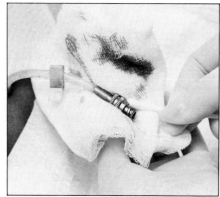

14 Use a sterile gauze pad to remove the tubing from the I.V. pole, and prepare to connect the tubing to the catheter. Remove the cap from the tubing. Then, connect the catheter to the tubing, and unclamp the catheter. Remove the drapes from the patient's lap, but leave the bed-saver pad in place.

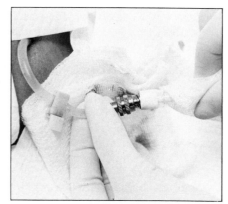

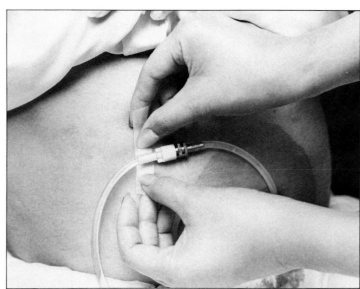

15 Now, tape the tubing to the patient's abdomen, as the nurse is doing here. Finally, open the roller clamp to begin draining dialysate into the patient's abdomen. When the dialysate's drained into her abdomen, have the patient fold the empty bag and replace it inside her clothing. (See the home care aid on pages 138 to 140 for the correct way to fold the bag.) Remove the bed-saver pad from your patient's lap and discard the equipment. Document the exchange on your patient's dialysis record and in your nurses' notes.

Patient teaching

Home care

How to perform a continuous ambulatory peritoneal dialysis (CAPD) solution exchange

1 Dear Patient:
You and your doctor have chosen continuous ambulatory peritoneal dialysis (CAPD) for your dialysis program. CAPD has an advantage over other forms of dialysis, because it's less expensive and easier to perform at home. But, it has a big disadvantage, too. If you use CAPD, you may get an infection in your abdomen. So, when performing a CAPD solution exchange at home, you must guard against harmful bacteria entering the dialysis system. The following instructions will tell you the best way to drain out the used dialysate and replace it with fresh dialysate, so that you don't contaminate the system.

First, gather the equipment you need: a 2-liter bag of peritoneal dialysis solution of the correct dextrose concentration; two outlet port clamps; and a sterile CAPD prep kit, which includes povidone-iodine swabs, 4"x4" sterile gauze pads, nonallergenic tape, and a mask. If you must inject medication into the dialysate, you'll also need the necessary number of 25G needles, 10 cc syringes, and the medication itself. Obtain an I.V. pole, if you have one.

Before you begin, warm the dialysate by placing it in a basin or sink full of warm water. Be sure the protective wrap remains on the bag and take care to keep the bag's ports dry. Remember to wash your hands thoroughly.

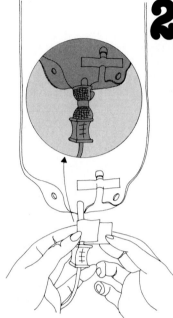

2 Open the CAPD prep kit. Then, remove the empty dialysate bag from inside your clothing. Tape the bag's injection port so it's out of the way. Before you open the junction of the bag and tubing spike, you must clean the junction. To do so, wrap a povidone-iodine-soaked swab around it. Then, wrap a dry gauze pad around the swab, and tape the gauze pad in position, as shown in the inset.

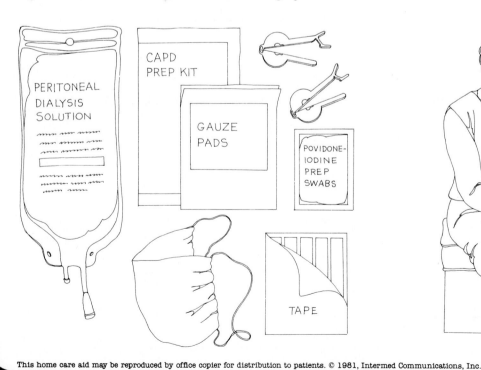

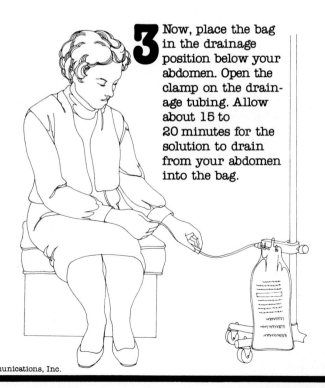

3 Now, place the bag in the drainage position below your abdomen. Open the clamp on the drainage tubing. Allow about 15 to 20 minutes for the solution to drain from your abdomen into the bag.

4 Meanwhile, remove the dialysate bag wrapping. Look at the dialysate solution to make sure it's clear, not cloudy. Also, read the concentration information on the label to make sure you have the right solution. Check the expiration date. Squeeze the bag firmly to test it for leaks.

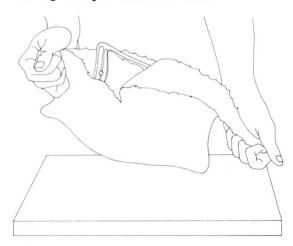

5 If your doctor's ordered it, add medication to the bag. To do so, first put on your mask. Draw up the medication and wipe the injection port with a povidone-iodine swab. Inject the needle through the rubber stopper into the injection port. To mix the dialysate and the medication, upend the bag several times.

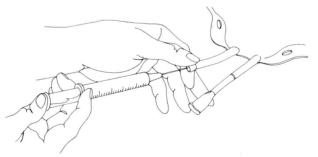

6 When the dialysate has finished draining from your abdomen, close the clamp and place the drainage bag on a flat surface, next to the new bag. Position the used dialysate bag with its clear side up so you can check the fluid for cloudiness or particles. Position the new dialysate bag with its label side up so you can double-check the dialysate concentration and expiration date. Arrange the bags so that their ends extend over the edge of the work surface.

Now, put on a mask, if you haven't done so already. Tape the injection port of the new bag to keep it from touching the outlet port. Place a clamp on the outlet port, to keep it stable during spike insertion.

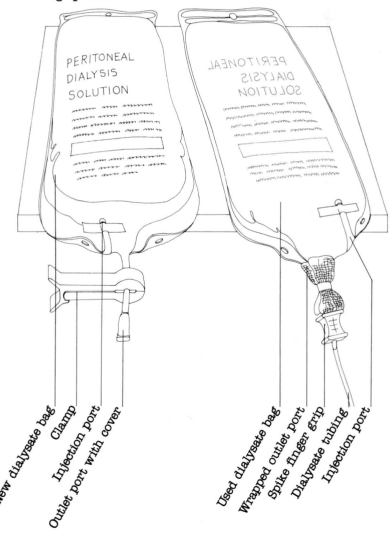

Patient teaching

Home care

How to perform a continuous ambulatory peritoneal dialysis (CAPD) solution exchange continued

7 Now, remove the gauze pads from the outlet-port tubing junction. Clamp the outlet port, lining up the clamp with the first step notch on the port.

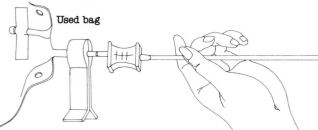

Used bag

8 Remove the blue covering from the outlet port of the new bag, without touching the port. Now, you're ready to transfer the tubing spike.

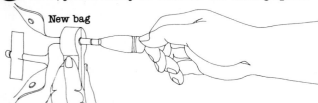

New bag

9 Grasp the finger grip on the tubing spike in the drainage-bag outlet port. With your free hand, hold the clamp on the outlet port. Twist and pull the spike to remove it from the port. *Take care not to touch anything with the spike tip.*

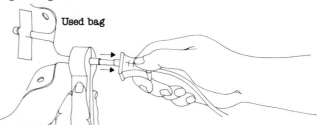

Used bag

10 Immediately insert the spike into the outlet port of the new bag. Unclamp the outlet port.

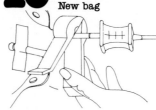

New bag

11 New bag

Hang the new bag on an I.V. pole. Then, open the clamp to allow the dialysate to drain into your abdomen. After about 5 minutes, when almost all the dialysate has drained from the bag, close the clamp. By leaving a little fluid in the bag, you will make the bag easier to fold.

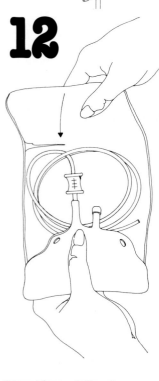

12 Remove the bag from the pole and place it in front of you. Fold over the spike-outlet port connection so it's centered on the bag. Coil the tubing over this connection. Then, fold the other end of the bag over the connection and tubing and place the bag inside a pouch, if you use one. Put the pouch inside your clothing. If your doctor's ordered a drainage sample, take the entire bag of fluid to the hospital lab for analysis. Otherwise, carefully empty the used dialysate into the toilet, and discard the empty bag in a trash can.

Home care

Continuous ambulatory peritoneal dialysis (CAPD) daily record

Name: _Mary Doe_   Date: _1-2-81_

Ideal weight: _147_ lbs.   Daily weight (after draining out third exchange): _150_ lbs.

Yesterday's weight: _148_ lbs. (Use daily weight from yesterday's record.)

Weight change (indicate plus or minus): _+2_ lbs.
(To find out your weight change, add or subtract today's daily weight from yesterday's.)

Temperature: _99°_   Pulse rate: _88_   Respiration rate: _20_

Blood pressure (standing up): _140/90_   Blood pressure (lying down): _130/86_

Catheter care: _Done — No swelling or tenderness around site_

1.5% dextrose solution	4.25% dextrose solution	Medications added	Solution in		Amount of fluid in (ml)	Solution out		Amount of fluid out (ml)	Fluid loss or gain (ml)
			Time started	Time finished		Time started	Time finished		
✓		None	7⁰⁰ AM	7¹⁰ AM	2000	2⁴⁰ PM	3⁰⁰ PM	2000	0
✓		None	3⁰⁰ PM	3¹⁰ PM	2000	10⁴⁰ PM	11⁰⁰ PM	1900	+100
	✓	None	11⁰⁰ PM	11¹⁰ PM	2000	6⁴⁰ AM	7⁰⁰ AM	2400	-400
									TOTAL
									-300

Comments: _Slight nausea this AM_
Lower back pain, all day

Dialysis

Nurses' guide to peritoneal dialysis complications

Complication	Possible causes	Nursing considerations
Peritonitis Indicated by fever, persistent abdominal pain and cramping, abdominal fullness, abdominal rigidity, slow dialysis drainage, inability to obtain a predialysis ascitic fluid specimen, cloudy drainage, swelling and tenderness around the catheter, and increased white blood cell count	• Poor aseptic technique during catheter insertion or dialysis	• Use scrupulous aseptic technique throughout entire dialysis procedure. • If you suspect peritonitis, notify the doctor immediately. He'll order continuous peritoneal dialysis and antibiotic therapy. • Send peritoneal fluid sample to lab for fluid analysis, culture and sensitivity, Gram's stain, and cell count.
Exit site infection Indicated by redness, swelling, rigidity, tenderness, and purulent drainage around catheter	• Poor aseptic technique during catheter insertion or dialysis • Incomplete healing around exit-site cuff of Tenckhoff catheter	• Use scrupulous aseptic technique throughout entire dialysis procedure. • Notify doctor immediately. He will order antibiotic therapy. • Obtain a culture of exit-site drainage and send it to lab.
Subcutaneous tunnel infection with Tenckhoff catheter Indicated by redness, rigidity, swelling, and tenderness over subcutaneous tunnel	• Poor aseptic technique during catheter insertion or dialysis • Incomplete healing in subcutaneous tunnel	• Use strict aseptic technique throughout entire dialysis procedure. • Notify doctor immediately. He will order antibiotic therapy.
Perforation of the bladder or bowel Indicated by peritonitis signs and symptoms; bright yellow dialysate drainage (if bladder is perforated), or feces in drainage (if bowel is perforated)	• Catheter inserted when patient had full bladder or bowel	• Have patient empty bladder and bowel before surgery. Doctor will order laxatives or catheterization, if necessary. • If you suspect perforation, notify doctor immediately.
Bleeding through catheter	• Minor trauma to the abdomen • Minor trauma to the subcutaneous tunnel (with Tenckhoff catheter) • Perforation of a major abdominal blood vessel during surgery	• Bleeding usually stops spontaneously. If not, notify the doctor, who may order blood transfusions or patient returned to the operating room. • Doctor may order 1,000 ml hourly dialysis exchanges, until drainage is clear.
Dialysate leakage around catheter	• Excessive instillation of dialysate	• Instill less dialysate at exchanges. Drain the patient's abdomen completely during outflow.
	• Incomplete healing around cuff of Tenckhoff catheter	• Doctor may order bed rest to permit healing. • Use small volumes of dialysate in exchanges through a new catheter. Also, drain the patient's abdomen completely during outflow.
	• Catheter obstruction	• Irrigate the catheter with sterile normal saline solution.
	• Catheter dislodged or improperly positioned	• Doctor must replace catheter or revise its position surgically.
Kinking of Tenckhoff catheter	• Subcutaneous tunnel too short • Scarring in the subcutaneous tunnel	• Doctor removes the catheter and implants a new one.
Lower back pain	• Pressure and weight of dialysate in abdomen, particularly in CAPD patients	• Doctor may order analgesics. • Doctor may order exercises to strengthen patient's muscles and improve his posture.

Complication	Possible causes	Nursing considerations
Abdominal or rectal pain (with possible referred pain in shoulder)	• Improperly positioned catheter tip causing irritation	• Doctor will revise catheter position surgically.
	• Dialysate accumulating under diaphragm	• Drain abdomen completely during outflow.
Ileus Indicated by sharp pain in abdomen, constipation, abdominal distention, nausea and vomiting, and diarrhea	• Catheter (especially Tenckhoff) manipulated excessively during insertion	• Notify the doctor immediately because signs and symptoms may indicate peritonitis. • Insert a nasogastric tube to suction patient, as ordered. • Administer medication, such as neostigmine (Prostigmin*) to relieve gas, as ordered. • Insert rectal tube to relieve distention. • Administer fluids and electrolytes I.V., as ordered. However, don't give patient anything to eat or drink. • Ambulate the patient, unless ordered otherwise by the doctor. • Prepare the patient for surgery, if the doctor orders. • Condition may spontaneously disappear after 12 hours.
Cramping	• Dialysate warmer or cooler than 98.6° F. (37° C.)	• Warm dialysate to 98.6° F. (37° C.) before infusion.
	• Rapid infusion or drainage	• Decrease infusion or drainage rate.
	• Pressure from excess dialysate in abdomen	• Infuse less dialysate at exchanges.
	• Chemical irritation	• Use dialysate with less than 7% dextrose concentration.
	• Air in abdomen	• Clamp off dialysate tubing before dialysate completely empties into abdomen.
Excessive fluid loss	• Use of dialysate with incorrect dextrose concentration • Inadequate sodium intake • Inadequate fluid intake	• Monitor patient's weight and blood pressure. • Be sure patient is receiving dialysate with correct dextrose concentration. Doctor may order reduced dextrose concentration. • Doctor will order increased fluid and sodium intake.
Fluid overload	• Use of dialysate with incorrect dextrose concentration • Excessive sodium intake • Excessive fluid intake	• Monitor patient's weight and blood pressure. • Doctor will order reduced fluid and sodium intake. • Doctor may order increased use of dialysate with 4.25% dextrose concentration.
Hernia (asymptomatic)	• In CAPD patients, increased abdominal pressure from nausea, vomiting, or constipation	• Observe patient for pain, discomfort, or abdominal rigidity. • Instruct patient to avoid overexertion. • Doctor will order medication to relieve nausea and vomiting, or to prevent constipation.

*Available in both the United States and in Canada

Renal transplant

Renal transplant. Not too long ago it was considered experimental. Now, about 3,000 end stage renal disease (ESRD) patients receive transplanted kidneys every year.

Most probably, you'll have to care for a renal transplant patient, if you haven't already. Do you know just what to do?

For example, can you recognize the signs of organ rejection? How will you prepare your patient for the procedures he'll undergo? Do you understand immunosuppressive therapy and its side effects?

To prepare yourself for these nursing challenges, study the information on the following pages.

Learning about renal transplants

After several years of dialysis, your patient has decided to have a renal transplant. Whatever his reason for deciding, he's not alone. Since the procedure first was performed more than 25 years ago, over 24,000 patients have decided, in consultation with their doctors, to have renal transplant surgery. About 45% of these patients still survive. Moreover, more than 300 women who received new kidneys later became pregnant and chose to give birth. They had healthy children who showed few adverse effects from the immunosuppressive medications their mothers took.

One of the major obstacles to a successful renal transplant is finding a suitable donor. Blood relatives make the most compatible donors. Transplanted kidneys donated by a patient's identical twin have approximately a 95% success rate. A kidney from any other sibling has about an 80% success rate. A parent-to-child transplant has approximately a 75% success rate.

However, most kidneys for transplant come from cadavers, although these kidneys pose a higher risk of rejection than living-related donor kidneys. On the average, cadaver kidneys have about a 50% success rate for the first year after surgery.

One serious complication of renal transplant surgery is that your patient may reject his transplanted kidney. Also, medications taken to suppress his immune system will increase his susceptibility to infection.

After surgery, your patient will need a high-protein diet to facilitate tissue healing. And, as long as he has the transplanted kidney, he'll take immunosuppressive drugs to help prevent rejection. Barring complications, or adverse side effects from the medications, a renal transplant patient can look forward to improved general health and a lifestyle free of dialysis equipment.

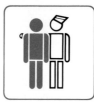

Preparing your patient for renal transplant surgery

How much does your patient understand about renal transplant surgery? To him, this probably will be a frightening and highly emotional experience. No doubt, he has mixed feelings about the surgery. He may be happy that a donor's available, but fearful of the surgery and its outcome. You can significantly lessen your patient's emotional turmoil by preparing him properly. To help, follow the guidelines on pages 74 and 75 for preparing a patient for urinary tract surgery. Here are some additional tips that apply for your renal transplant patient:

• Encourage your patient to express his feelings. Is he worried that his body will reject the new kidney? Perhaps he's afraid of what will happen to him in the recovery room. When you know what's worrying him, you can help him overcome his fears.

• Remind your patient that he'll undergo dialysis before surgery to rid him of excess fluid and electrolytes. Also, mention the possibility that he'll need dialysis after surgery if the new kidney doesn't function immediately.

• Instruct your patient not to smoke. Smoking may cause postoperative pulmonary complications.

• Explain the routine preoperative procedures your patient will undergo; for example, chest X-ray, electrocardiogram (EKG), enema, and shaving of the operative area. Also, tell your patient that he will not be allowed to eat or drink after midnight on the night before surgery. Be sure your patient understands the importance of blood-crossmatching and tissue-compatibility tests and how they will help ensure his body's acceptance of the new kidney.

• Tell your patient what to expect when he awakes from the anesthesia. Prepare him for any postoperative pain. Tell him pain medication will be available if he needs it. Describe the recovery room and its procedures, including the need for frequent vital-sign checks, respiratory care, and regulation of intravenous intake and urine output. Explain the other tubes and equipment and their functions. Include the urethral catheter, arterial line, and respirator. If your hospital permits, take your patient on a preoperative tour of the recovery room and intensive-care unit.

• Instruct your patient in the proper procedure for postoperative turning, coughing, and diaphragmatic breathing. Also, if ordered, teach him how to use an incentive spirometer. (For help in teaching these procedures, see the NURSING PHOTOBOOK PROVIDING RESPIRATORY CARE.)

• Finally, talk to your patient about the possible rejection of his new kidney. Reassure him that acute rejection is common and can be reversed. Also, discuss the immunosuppressive medications he'll be taking and their possible side effects. Warn your patient that these medications will increase his susceptibility to infection. Because of this, he must temporarily remain in his hospital room or be kept in reverse isolation.

Helping the donor

With all the care and attention the renal transplant recipient receives, the donor may feel left out or neglected. Remember, the donor needs the same preparation and emotional support. He'll be undergoing many of the same laboratory tests and will have similar questions about what to expect after surgery. Follow the same guidelines listed on the opposite page to prepare the donor.

In addition, you'll want to consider the psychological impact donating a kidney may have. Here are some tips:

• Offer emotional support to the donor and his family. Encourage them to talk openly about their concerns.

• Prepare the donor to deal with the possibility that his kidney may be physiologically rejected by the recipient. Explain that this happens occasionally and doesn't mean his kidney was inadequate.

• Refer the donor and his family for counseling, if they have not been counseled already.

Preserving a cadaver kidney

Will your patient receive a cadaver kidney? Most kidneys for renal transplant come from cadavers rather than from living-related donors. Do you know how a suitable cadaver's found?

Most cadavers have suffered fatal head trauma. Therefore, their availability can't be predicted. For a cadaver to be used for renal transplant, the donor must be diagnosed legally brain dead and may be artificially sustained on a respirator. Also, he must have been less than 55 years old, and free of infection, renal disease, hypertension, and cancer.

If the cadaver meets these conditions, it's tested for compatibility with the renal transplant patient. Provided the tests prove favorable, a surgeon will remove the kidney from the cadaver and place it in a preservation machine, like the one shown in this photograph. This machine keeps the kidney healthy by pumping plasma and oxygen into it. A temperature of 43° to 46.5° F. (6° to 8° C.) is maintained inside the machine.

Even with this machine, however, a cadaver kidney can be maintained for only 72 hours after it's removed from the donor. That's why the recipient usually undergoes renal transplant surgery within 24 hours after a suitable cadaver/donor is found.

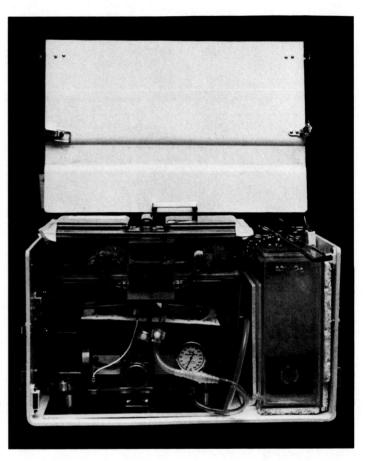

Understanding preoperative procedures

Your patient's decided to have renal transplant surgery. A donor's available. Now, the series of preoperative procedures begin. Do you know what these procedures include?

To begin, the doctor will evaluate your patient's general health to make sure he can undergo surgery. He'll also assess the condition of the patient's urinary tract to rule out ureteral reflux or a bladder infection. In some cases, the doctor will remove the patient's spleen to help the patient tolerate immunosuppressive medications and lessen the risk of rejection.

The doctor will also order many blood tests; for example, a complete blood count (CBC), paying particular attention to the white blood cell (WBC) count. Record the preoperative WBC value and monitor subsequent values closely. An elevated WBC after surgery may signal infection or rejection of the new kidney.

In addition, you'll need to determine your patient's fluid and electrolyte levels. Remember, renal failure patients usually have elevated electrolyte levels. After surgery, these levels should return to normal. Record blood urea nitrogen (BUN), serum creatinine, calcium, and phosphorus values, too, if ordered. Be sure to notify the doctor immediately if you detect significant changes in any subsequent blood values.

Probably the most important series of tests will determine the patient's and donor's blood type, antigen, and lymphocyte compatibility. These critical tests, listed below, help ensure that your patient will accept the transplanted kidney:

• **Human leukocyte antigen (HLA):** The HLA test determines compatibility between the donor's and patient's antigens. The greater the compatibility, the better the chance the kidney will be accepted.

• **Mixed lymphocyte culture (MLC):** White blood cells from the patient and the donor are combined in a test tube and incubated for 5 days. The results show how the patient's and donor's cells react together. A negative reaction indicates compatibility. *Note:* This test is performed only with a living-related donor.

• **Blood typing and crossmatching:** These tests determine the patient's and donor's blood compatibility. If their blood isn't compatible, the patient will reject the new kidney. For more details on blood typing and crossmatching, see the NURSING PHOTOBOOK MANAGING I.V. THERAPY.

Renal transplant

Patient preparation

Does your patient have questions about the surgical procedure he'll undergo when he receives a new kidney? If so, show him the illustration to the right and explain it in these easily understandable terms:

Tell him he'll be taken to the operating room (OR) and given anesthesia. After he's asleep, the surgeon will make an incision on the patient's side like the one in the illustration. The patient's nonfunctioning kidneys will probably be left in place. If removal was indicated, the surgeon would have done it several weeks before the renal transplant surgery.

Meanwhile, the donor will undergo a similar surgical procedure in an adjacent operating room. (If a cadaver donor's used, the kidney will be in a preservation machine, as explained on page 145.)

Note: If the donor's left kidney is used, the surgeon will place it in the patient's right side. The opposite is true if the donor's right kidney is used. This positioning permits the renal pelvis to rest anteriorly. It also allows the new kidney's ureter to rest in front of the iliac artery, where the ureter's more accessible.

Next, the new kidney's placed in the hollow of the patient's hip bone (see illustration). The surgeon connects the new kidney's renal artery to the patient's hypogastric artery. Then, he'll connect the new kidney's renal vein to the recipient's external iliac vein. He'll also attach the new kidney's ureter to the patient's bladder. When the transplant's complete, the surgeon sutures the incision closed and sends the patient to the recovery room. The surgery takes about 4 hours.

Postoperative assessment and care

The transplant surgery has been completed and your patient has returned to the transplant unit. Now, you're responsible for giving him the proper postoperative care. Do you know how?

You must recognize the complications that may occur after renal transplant surgery. These complications include:
- bacterial, viral, or other systemic infections
- wound infection, lymphocele, or hematoma
- renal artery stenosis, thrombosis, or aneurysm
- urologic obstruction, leak, or fistula
- side effects caused by immunosuppressive medications.

Most important, remember you're caring for a chronically ill patient whose immune system has been suppressed by medication. Consequently, he runs a much higher risk of infection. To lessen the risk, use strict aseptic technique when changing his dressings or caring for his catheter. (For more details, see pages 84 and 85.)

Also, restrict his contact with other patients in the unit and with visitors. Ask your patient's visitors to wear surgical masks for the first 2 weeks after surgery. If your patient's white blood cell (WBC) count falls below 2,000 cells/mm³, the doctor may isolate him. If so, restrict visitors to the immediate family and follow your hospital's isolation policy. Also, limit the number of nurses who come in contact with the patient. Any nurse or visitor with an upper respiratory infection should wear a surgical mask whenever he comes in contact with the patient.

Of course, you'll begin your care with a thorough assessment. This illustration shows you what you need to include in your assessment and lists the appropriate nursing actions.

1 FLUID AND ELECTROLYTES
Nursing action
- Frequently monitor vital signs, especially blood pressure. Increased blood pressure may indicate fluid retention; decreased blood pressure may indicate hypovolemic shock. Note possible effects of any preoperative antihypertensive therapy.
- Note any blood or plasma volume expanders your patient received. Make sure blood is available for transfusions, if needed.
- Monitor fluid and electrolyte levels. Report abnormal levels and prepare to treat condition, as ordered.
- Weigh patient daily to check for excessive fluid retention. Report to the doctor a weight increase or decrease of more than 3 pounds (1.4 kg) in one day.
- Replace urine output with I.V. fluid, if ordered.
- Check dressing for excessive incisional bleeding, and record estimated drainage as output.

2 PULMONARY
Nursing action
- Check respirations.
- Be sure patient follows postoperative coughing and deep-breathing exercises. Also, have patient use incentive spirometer, if ordered.

3 CARDIAC
Nursing action
- Monitor EKG and compare with previous readings.
- Check pulse frequently. *Note:* tachycardia may indicate hypovolemic shock. Cardiac arrhythmias may indicate potassium imbalance.
- Check frequently for signs of congestive heart failure and pulmonary edema.
- Be sure patient's placed on cardiac monitor and X-rays are ordered to check for cardiac enlargement.

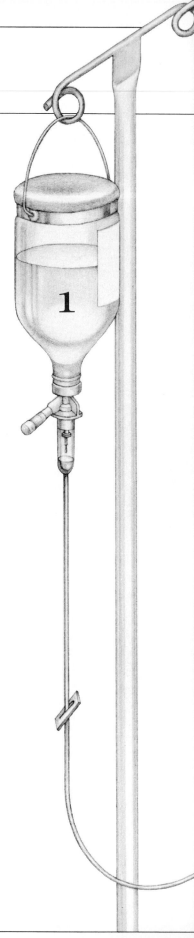

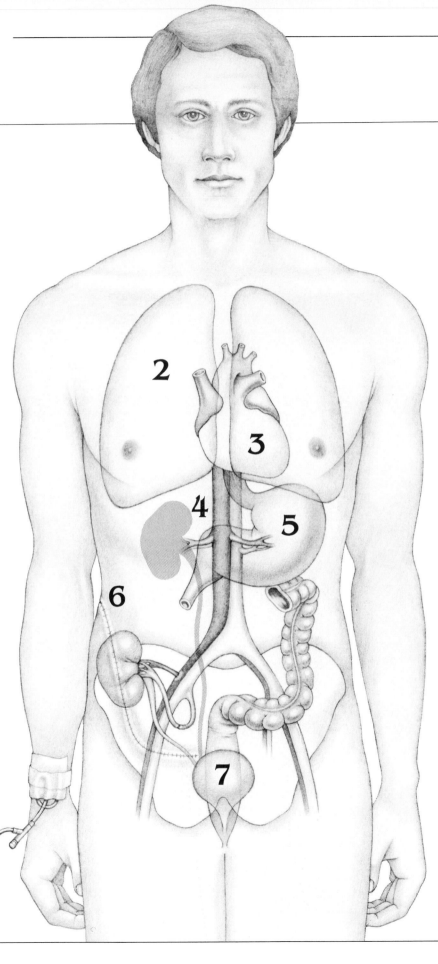

4 ARTERIOVENOUS CIRCULATION

Nursing action
• Check patency of intravenous lines, including arterial line. (For more details, see NURSING PHOTOBOOK USING MONITORS.) Also, check patency of peripheral intravenous lines. (For more details, see NURSING PHOTOBOOK MANAGING I.V. THERAPY.)
• Inspect color, warmth, and movement of patient's extremities, especially the leg on his operative side.
• Observe patient's level of consciousness.
• Check for bruit and thrill at vascular access site.

5 GASTROINTESTINAL

Nursing action
• Check bowel sounds. If none are present, notify the doctor. The patient may have a paralytic ileus.
• Check nasogastric tube, if inserted. Be sure the suction machine's working properly. Watch for signs of bowel or nasogastric tube obstruction.

6 WOUND CARE

Nursing action
• Maintain aseptic technique when caring for a wound. Clean suture line daily with povidone-iodine solution and apply povidone-iodine ointment.
• Report any signs of infection, including redness, swelling, purulent drainage, turgidity, warmth or pain around wound. These signs also may indicate rejection of the transplanted kidney.
• Check wound and dressing for excessive bleeding. Also check wound for evisceration or dehiscence, as explained on page 101.
• Empty the Jackson-Pratt suction reservoir at least once every 4 hours. Record amount of drainage. (For details, see page 148.)
• For the first 3 days postop, turn patient only on his back and operative side to minimize strain on anastomosed artery, vein, and ureter.
• Consider the effects of immunosuppressive medication, if healing seems slow.

7 UROLOGIC

Nursing action
• Measure urine output hourly. Report any significant increase or decrease to the doctor.
• Note catheter's patency and condition of insertion site. Perform catheter care every 8 hours. If blood clots are present, irrigate the catheter with normal saline solution, if ordered. (For more details, see pages 81 to 83).
• If the patient becomes anuric, irrigate the catheter for possible blood clots, as ordered. If no clots appear, notify the doctor.
• In your nurses' notes, describe the color, consistency, pH, and specific gravity of the urine.
• Remember, the patient may be oliguric immediately after surgery. This is common and may continue for several days.

Renal transplant

Using a Jackson-Pratt suction reservoir

1 *Does your patient have a Jackson-Pratt suction reservoir to drain postoperative fluid? In most cases, the reservoir and drain tube (shown in the inset) will be attached to the patient in the operating room. But, you'll need to empty it every 4 hours and re-dress the wound. Do you know how?*

Obtain this equipment: a graduated container, Betadine ointment, gauze pad, a Surgipad, sterile gloves, and nonallergenic adhesive tape.

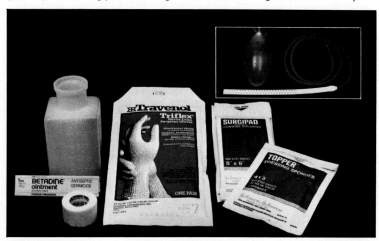

2 Before you begin, tell your patient what you're going to do and reassure her that she'll feel no pain.

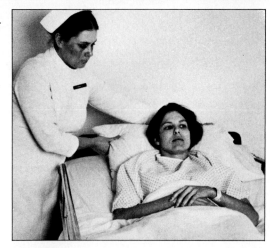

3 Now you're ready to empty the reservoir. Unpin the reservoir from your patient's gown. Grasp the tab on the reservoir and open the plug, as shown here.

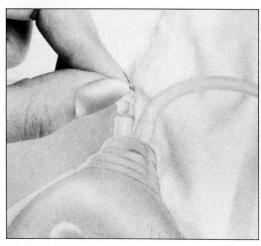

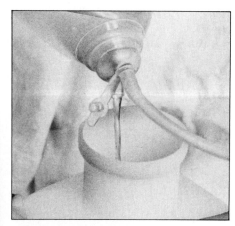

4 Next, pour the drained fluid into the graduated container. Note the amount of fluid.

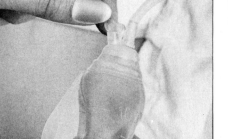

5 Squeeze the reservoir and replace its tab.

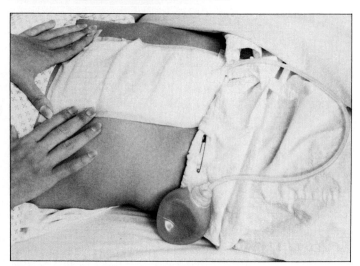

6 Repin the reservoir to your patient's gown. Finally, apply Betadine ointment to the wound. Using aseptic technique, re-dress the wound with a gauze pad and Surgipad. (For more details on re-dressing a wound, see pages 84 and 85.)

Document the entire procedure, including the amount, color, and odor of the drainage, in your nurses' notes. Also, record the amount of drainage on the patient's fluid input/output record.

Note: The Jackson-Pratt suction reservoir featured here is manufactured by the American Heyer-Schulte Corporation.

Recognizing rejection

As you know, one of the most serious complications that may occur after renal transplant surgery is that your patient's body will reject the newly transplanted kidney. *Remember:* The longer your patient keeps his new kidney, the less likely he'll be to reject it. But, the risk of rejection's always present.

Notify the doctor immediately if you notice any of these signs of rejection:
- redness, swelling, and tenderness over the transplant site
- elevated temperature

- elevated white blood cell (WBC) count
- decreased urine output
- increased proteinuria
- sudden weight gain
- simultaneously elevated serum creatinine and blood urea nitrogen (BUN) levels
- acute onset of hypertension
- sodium retention (puffy eyes, weight gain, and swollen extremities) only when accompanied by one or more of the other signs and symptoms listed above.

Understanding renal rejection

How well do you understand the three types of rejection that may occur after renal transplant surgery? Can you explain them to your patient? Most important, do you know what to do if rejection occurs? Study this chart to familiarize yourself with these complications.

Type of rejection	Time of occurrence	Description	Nursing intervention
Hyperacute	Within a few minutes to several hours after surgery	Patient's circulating antibodies attack kidney, drastically reducing blood flow to kidney. The kidney then becomes ischemic and dies. Hyperacute rejection is irreversible.	• Prepare patient for surgery to remove rejected kidney, if indicated. • Give emotional support to help lessen patient's disappointment and aid his adjustment. • If indicated, provide emotional support to donor, who may think that he has failed.
Acute	With living-related donor, from first week after surgery to 6 months. With cadaver donor, from first week after surgery to 1 year	The new kidney secretes antigens into the patient's blood serum where they're recognized as foreign. The patient's immune system is activated and produces a specific antibody. Then, the antibody attacks the new kidney's cells. Acute rejection is reversible.	• Report signs of rejection to the doctor. (See *Danger Signs* on this page.) • Prepare patient for renal blood flow scan. • Observe for signs of systemic and wound infection. Signs of systemic infection include elevated temperature, rapid pulse, lethargy, and elevated white blood cell (WBC) count. (See page 101 for the signs of wound infection.) • Monitor blood pressure frequently for hypertension. • Weigh patient frequently. A weight gain of more than 3 pounds (1.4 kg) may indicate fluid retention. Notify the doctor if this occurs. • Reassure patient that acute rejection is common and reversible. Also, teach him to recognize the possible side effects of immunosuppressive medications. (For details, see pages 150 and 151.)
Chronic	Anytime after surgery	Glomerular filtration rates decrease gradually. Blood urea nitrogen (BUN) and serum creatinine rise progressively. Chronic rejection is a long-term response to the transplanted kidney and is irreversible.	• Reassure patient that chronic rejection is a slow process and can take many years before complete renal function is lost. • Give support to family members. • Prepare patient for renal biopsy, if ordered. • Check blood pressure frequently to observe for hypertension. • Prepare patient for dialysis, if indicated. • Administer increased immunosuppressive medication, if ordered. • Monitor patient's weight. Excessive weight gain may indicate fluid retention. Notify doctor. • Frequently monitor results of renal and other laboratory studies. • Adjust diet and fluid regimen, if ordered. • Prepare patient for additional dialysis treatments, or another transplant, if indicated.

Renal transplant

Understanding immunosuppressive procedures

For renal transplant surgery to be successful, the doctor must implement some special procedures to prevent the patient's body from rejecting the new kidney. These immunosuppressive procedures suppress the body's immune system.

One way the doctor may suppress your patient's immune system is with medication. You can learn more about these immunosuppressive medications by studying the chart on these pages.

The doctor may also order one or several other procedures to lessen the risk of rejection. Here's how these procedures work:

• **Radiation therapy** destroys peripheral lymphocytes and prevents antibody formation. Only the transplant site is irradiated. Assure your patient that he'll receive only a small dose of radiation.

• **Total lymphoid irradiation** weakens or destroys the lymph nodes' ability to reject the new kidney. All lymph nodes in the patient's abdomen, chest, and arms are exposed to radiation.

• **Spleenectomy** decreases the number of circulating lymphocytes by eliminating the spleen, where they're produced. Some doctors believe that removing the spleen also improves the patient's tolerance of azathioprine (Imuran*), an immunosuppressive drug. Unfortunately, a spleenectomy may cause thromboembolic complications.

• **Thoracic duct lymph drainage** allows the doctor to drain the lymphatic fluid. After he drains the fluid, the lab will freeze it and discard the lymphocytes. The remaining lymphatic fluid is then transfused into the patient. This method decreases the patient's cellular immunity response. However, it can increase the chance of septicemia.

Nurses' guide to immunosuppressive drugs

As you know, your patient will need immunosuppressive drugs for as long as he has a transplanted kidney. Without this medication, his body will recognize the kidney as a foreign body and reject it.

Here's a chart of the most common immunosuppressive drugs. Remember, the doctor will adjust all dosages according to the patient's needs.

Refer to the NURSE'S GUIDE TO DRUGS™ for more information about these and other drugs your patient may be receiving.

Important: Because of your patient's increased susceptibility to infection, limit the number of nurses who come in contact with him. Also, observe him carefully for signs of infection, such as fever or sore throat.

Drug	Indication and dosage	
azathioprine Imuran*	*Immunosuppressive agent* **Adults:** Initially, 3 to 5 mg/kg P.O. daily. Maintain at 1 to 2 mg/kg/day.	
cyclophosphamide Cytoxan*	*Antineoplastic administered when Imuran causes hepatotoxicity* **Adults:** 40 to 50 mg/kg, P.O., I.V., in single dose or in 2 to 8 daily doses; then adjust for maintenance.	
methylprednisolone sodium succinate Solu-Medrol*	*Immunosuppressive agent* **Adults:** 2 to 60 mg P.O. in 4 divided doses; or 10 to 250 mg I.M. or I.V. every 4 hours	
prednisone Deltasone*	*Immunosuppressive agent* **Adults:** 2.5 to 15 mg P.O., b.i.d., t.i.d., or q.i.d.	

*Available in both the United States and in Canada

Possible side effects	Special considerations
Drug-induced hepatitis, acute pancreatitis, leukopenia, skin rash, increased risk of infection, bone marrow depression, hepatotoxicity, anorexia, nausea, vomiting, steatorrhea, mouth ulceration, alopecia, thrombocytopenia, anemia	• If patient received cadaver kidney, doctor may reduce dosage because of delayed renal function. • Observe for signs of liver toxicity, clay-colored stools, dark urine, pruritus, yellow skin or sclera. • Monitor bilirubin level and complete blood cell (CBC) count to check for hepatotoxicity. • Administer antiemetic to reduce nausea and vomiting, if ordered. • If patient has steatorrhea, administer medication to control it, if ordered. • Warn patient to report even mild infection; for example, sore throat.
Leukopenia, thrombocytopenia, anemia, anorexia, nausea, vomiting, stomatitis, sterility, bone marrow depression, thrombophlebitis, potassium depletion, hemorrhagic cystitis, alopecia, buccal irritation, increased risk of infection	• Give antiemetic before administering drug to reduce nausea and vomiting, if ordered. • Warn patient that alopecia is likely to occur. • Observe patient for signs of bleeding and bruising. • Have patient report any leg pain or cramping. • Encourage adequate diet and fluid intake. • Give mouth care to prevent ulcerations. • Monitor electrolyte levels, CBC, and renal function studies. • Avoid I.M. administration. • Warn patient to avoid contact with contagious diseases.
Headache, depression, convulsions, hypertension, congestive heart failure, cataracts, perforated ulcer, Cushing's syndrome (round cheeks, protruding abdomen, fat deposits over upper back, acne, increased facial and body hair), delayed wound healing, petechiae, suppressed growth in children, menstrual abnormalities, muscle weakness, increased infection risk, herpes outbreak, negative nitrogen balance, anaphylaxis with circulatory collapse, musculoskeletal defects, increased intracranial pressure, fluid and electrolyte imbalance, adrenal insufficiency, osteoporosis *Withdrawal symptoms:* Rebound inflammation, fatigue, weakness, arthralgia, fever, dizziness, lethargy, depression, dyspnea, hypoglycemia, hypotension	• Gradually reduce dosage after long-term therapy. Sudden withdrawal of drug may be fatal. • Increase dosage, as ordered, during stress. • Also, teach patient signs of adrenal insufficiency caused by sudden withdrawal of drug or increased stress. • Warn patient not to discontinue drug suddenly and teach him to recognize signs of drug withdrawal. • Monitor patient's weight, blood pressure, and serum electrolyte levels. • Administer drug with food, if possible. • Give I.V. doses slowly to prevent arrhythmias or circulatory collapse. • Discard reconstituted solutions after 48 hours. • When mixing Solu-Medrol, use only diluent accompanying vial. • If patient is diabetic, increase insulin dosage, if ordered, while administering this drug. Monitor blood sugar frequently. • Avoid administering aspirin. • Provide low-sodium, high-potassium diet. • Warn patient to avoid contact with contagious diseases. • Treat wounds immediately.
Convulsions, headache, Cushing's syndrome, increased appetite, mood swings, delayed wound healing, increased infection risk, cataracts, perforated ulcer, edema, steroid-induced diabetes mellitus, hypertension, negative nitrogen balance, congestive heart failure, menstrual abnormalities, fluid and electrolyte level imbalance, myopathies, osteoporosis, muscle atrophy, pathologic fracture *Withdrawal symptoms:* See methylprednisolone sodium succinate.	• Gradually reduce drug dosage after long-term therapy. Sudden withdrawal of drug may be fatal. • Weigh patient daily and report any sudden weight gain to doctor. • Monitor blood pressure. • Monitor serum electrolyte levels. • Administer drug with food. • Give antacids, if ordered. • Provide low-sodium, high-potassium, and high-protein diet. • Avoid administering aspirin. • Watch for depression or psychotic episodes. • Teach patient to recognize side effects and signs of adrenal insufficiency. • Increase dosage during stress, if ordered. • Warn patient to avoid contact with contagious diseases. • Treat wounds immediately.

Patient teaching

Home care

How to take an accurate blood pressure measurement

1 Dear Family Member:
Because a member of your family has had a kidney transplant, you've been instructed to monitor his blood pressure daily. Before you begin, gather the equipment shown here: a blood pressure cuff with aneroid dial, and a stethoscope.

Note: Ask the nurse to fill in your family member's predetermined number here: _____

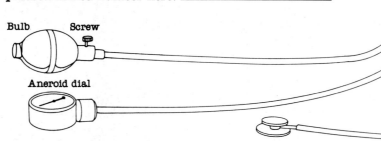

Bulb Screw

Aneroid dial

Blood pressure cuff

Earpieces

Stethoscope

Diaphragm

2 Use his brachial pulse to obtain a blood pressure measurement. To find this pulse, place your index and middle fingers in the crook of his arm. Feel for a beat.

Important: Ask him to relax for 5 minutes before you begin so the measurement will be accurate. Also, be sure he's always in the same position, either sitting, standing, or reclining, unless the doctor directs otherwise.

Next, place his arm level with his heart, as shown here. Wrap the blood pressure cuff around his arm, as shown in the illustration. The cuff's lower edge should be at least 1″ (2.5 cm) above the pulse. To ensure an accurate reading, never apply the cuff over clothing.

Wrap the cuff securely so you can slide only two fingers between it and his arm. Place the aneroid dial where you can easily see it.

Now, place the tips of the stethoscope's earpieces in your ears. Be sure they're angled forward. Place the stethoscope's diaphragm over his brachial pulse.

Hold the bulb and turn the screw clockwise until it's closed. Squeeze the bulb quickly until the aneroid dial reaches his predetermined number.

Now, slowly release the screw counterclockwise. When you hear the first beating sound, note the number on the aneroid dial. This is his *systolic* pressure, or the top number of his blood pressure reading. Continue slowly deflating the cuff. When the beating stops, again note the number. This is his *diastolic* pressure, or the bottom number of his blood pressure reading.

When you're sure the beating has stopped completely, you can deflate the cuff quickly until the aneroid needle reads zero. Then, remove the cuff.

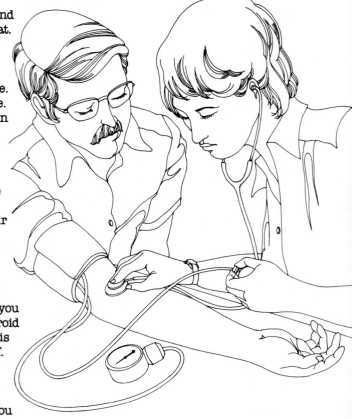

Home care

Going home after renal transplant surgery

Dear Patient:

Now that you're ready to go home, you'll need to follow these instructions to speed your recovery and help ensure that your new kidney functions properly. Here's what to do:

• Take medications exactly as your doctor orders. You must take these medications for as long as you have your transplanted kidney, so your body won't reject it. Never skip a dose or alter it in any way. If you forget or can't take your medication for any reason, call your doctor at once. Follow these special instructions:_____

_____

_____

_____

_____

_____

_____

Remember to take an antacid immediately before taking your medication. Also, avoid taking nonprescription drugs, such as aspirin or Tylenol, unless ordered by your doctor.

• Avoid overeating, even if you find your appetite has increased because of the medication you're taking. Excess weight can be harmful. For this reason, eat three well-balanced, calorie-controlled meals each day. Include high-protein foods, such as eggs, lean meats, fish, cheese, and skim milk. Avoid foods high in fat or carbohydrates. If you must snack, choose low-calorie, nutritious foods, such as fresh fruit.

• Drink four 8-oz. glasses of fluid each day, unless your doctor directs otherwise.

• Take your temperature every morning as soon as you awake. If your temperature goes above 100° F. (37.8° C.), call your doctor.

• Weigh yourself every morning before dressing. If you gain more than 3 pounds (1.4 kg) from one day to the next, call your doctor.

• Take your blood pressure twice each day, or ask a family member to take it for you. To ensure an accurate measurement, take it at the same time of day. Be sure you're in the same position each time, either sitting up, lying down, or standing. Remember to rest for at least 5 minutes before taking the measurement so your blood pressure can stabilize.

• Measure and record the amount of urine you produce in a 24-hour period. To do this, urinate into a container. Measure and record the amount. Then, discard the urine. If you urinate during the night, measure this, too. At the end of 24 hours, total the amount of urine you produced. Notify the doctor if your output is below 20 oz. (600 ml) during any 24-hour period.

• In a notebook, record your daily temperature, weight, blood pressure, and urine output. Bring this record with you to the doctor.

• See your doctor as frequently as he directs. Keep each appointment and follow your doctor's instructions exactly. Your next appointment's scheduled on:

_____

at _____o'clock.

You'll need to have eye examinations every 6 months for glaucoma and cataracts. Before you schedule a visit to the dentist, contact your doctor.

• Wait 6 weeks after surgery before engaging in sexual intercourse. Pregnancy poses an additional risk to your new kidney, so if you're female, practice a reliable birth-control method.

• Wait at least 2 weeks after returning home before you drive a car. Avoid wearing seat belts that may press on your new kidney. If you must wear a seat belt, wear it loosely.

• Exercise moderately. Begin slowly and increase the amount of exercise gradually. During the first 3 months after surgery, avoid excessive bending, heavy lifting, or contact sports, such as football.

• Avoid large groups of people during the first 3 months after surgery, to decrease the risk of contracting a contagious disease. Remember, your resistance to infection has been lowered by the medications you're taking.

Finally, call your doctor immediately if you notice any of these signs:

• redness, swelling, warmth, or tenderness over the new kidney

• fever over 100° F. (37.8° C.)

• decreased urine output

• blood pressure above _____

• sudden weight gain of more than 3 pounds (1.4 kg), or puffy eyelids and swollen ankles

• general feeling of uneasiness.

Appendix

Nurses' guide to bladder medications

Drug	Indications and dosage	Side effects	Contraindications
methenamine hippurate Hiprex (Hip-Rex in Canada)	*Long-term prophylaxis or suppression of chronic urinary tract infections* **Adults and children over age 12:** 1 gm taken orally every 12 hours **Children ages 6 to 12:** 500 mg to 1 gm taken orally every 12 hours	*Applies to all methenamine drugs:* Nausea; rashes; with high doses, urinary tract irritation, dysuria, urinary frequency, albuminuria, hematuria	*Applies to all methenamine drugs:* ● Renal insufficiency, severe liver disease, or severe dehydration
methenamine mandelate Mandelamine*	*Urinary tract infections, infected residual urine in patients with neurogenic bladder* **Adults:** 1 gm taken orally 4 times daily after meals **Children under age 6:** 50 mg/kg daily, divided into 4 doses, taken orally after meals **Children ages 6 to 12:** 500 mg taken orally 4 times daily after meals		
methenamine sulfosalicylate Hexalet	*Long-term prophylaxis or suppression of chronic urinary tract infections* **Adults and children over age 12:** 1 gm taken orally 4 times daily after meals with ½ glass of water **Children ages 6 to 12:** 500 mg taken orally 4 times daily after meals with ½ glass of water		
ascorbic acid (vitamin C) Ce-Vi-Sol*	*Urine acidification to potentiate methenamine effects* **Adults:** 100 mg taken orally 4 times daily **Children ages 6 to 12:** 50 to 100 mg daily, taken orally	Diarrhea, epigastric distress, oxaluria, renal stones	None
bethanechol chloride Urecholine*	*Acute postop and postpartum nonobstructive (functional) urinary retention, neurogenic atony of urinary bladder with retention* **Adults:** 50 to 100 mg taken orally 3 to 4 times daily	Lacrimation, excessive salivation, flushing, bronchoconstriction, abdominal cramps, nausea, vomiting, diarrhea, bradycardia or tachycardia, hypotension, increased perspiration	● In patients with weakened bladder wall ● When increased muscular activity of GI or urinary tract is harmful ● In mechanical obstructions of GI or urinary tract ● Hyperthyroidism, peptic ulcer, latent or active bronchial asthma, cardiac or coronary artery disease, vagotonia, epilepsy, Parkinson's disease, bradycardia, chronic obstructive pulmonary disease (COPD), hypotension, hypertension, pregnancy, vasomotor instability, peritonitis or other acute inflammatory conditions of GI tract
propantheline bromide Pro-Banthine*	*Neurogenic bladder—induces urinary retention, prevents bladder spasms* **Adults:** 15 mg taken orally twice daily before meals and 30 mg at bedtime, up to 60 mg 4 times daily. Or, with prolonged-action tablets, 30 mg taken orally every 8 to 12 hours, depending on individual response **Elderly adults:** 7.5 mg taken orally twice daily before meals. When oral dosage is not possible, give 30 mg I.M. or I.V. every 6 hours. *Maintenance dose* 15 mg I.M. every 6 hours	Blurred vision, drowsiness, dizziness, dry mouth, dysphagia, constipation, palpitations, tachycardia, urticaria, decreased perspiration, confusion or excitement in elderly patients	● Narrow-angle glaucoma, obstructive uropathy, obstructive disease of GI tract, severe ulcerative colitis, myasthenia gravis, hypersensitivity to anti-cholinergic drugs, paralytic ileus, intestinal atony, unstable cardiovascular status in acute hemorrhage, toxic megacolon ● Cautiously in autonomic neuropathy, hyperthyroidism, coronary heart disease, cardiac arrhythmias, congestive heart failure, hypertension, hiatal hernia associated with reflux esophagitis, hepatic or renal disease, ulcerative colitis, or patients over age 40 (because of the increased risk of glaucoma) ● Cautiously in hot or humid environments, because of increased risk of drug-induced heat stroke
oxybutynin chloride Ditropan	*Neurogenic bladder—induces urinary retention, prevents bladder spasms* **Adults:** 5 mg taken orally 2 to 3 times daily to a maximum of 5 mg 4 times daily **Children over age 5:** 5 mg taken orally twice daily to maximum of 5 mg 3 times daily.	Dry mouth, transient blurred vision, decreased perspiration, fever, drowsiness, dizziness, palpitations, tachycardia, nausea, vomiting, constipation, bloating, urticaria	● Obstructive uropathy, glaucoma, myasthenia gravis, GI obstruction, adynamic ileus, megacolon, severe or ulcerative colitis ● In elderly or debilitated patients with intestinal atony ● Cautiously with elderly patients and patients with autonomic neuropathy, reflex esophagitis, or hepatic or renal disease

*Available in both the United States and in Canada

Acknowledgements

Nursing considerations

Applies to all methenamine drugs:
• Oral suspension contains vegetable oil. Administer cautiously to elderly or debilitated patients because aspiration could cause lipid pneumonia.
• Limit intake of alkaline foods, such as vegetables, milk, peanuts, fruits, and fruit juices (except cranberry, plum, and prune juices, which may be used to acidify urine). Warn patient not to take antacids, including Alka-Seltzer® and other antacids containing sodium bicarbonate. Maintain urine pH at 5.5 or less. Use Nitrazine paper to check urine pH.
• If rash appears, withhold dose and contact doctor.
• Administer after meals to lessen GI upset.

• May inactivate orally administered penicillin G

• Never give I.M. or I.V. or you could cause circulatory collapse, hypotension, gastrointestinal distress, shock, or cardiac arrest.
• Because effective bladder-control dosage is high, watch closely for side effects that may indicate drug toxicosis. If you see any, call doctor promptly.
• After administering, monitor vital signs frequently, being especially careful to check respiration. Position patient to make breathing easier. Be prepared to give atropine 0.5 to 1 mg slow I.V. push, and provide respiratory support, if needed.
• Give drug on an empty stomach; if taken after meals, it may cause nausea and vomiting.

• Give 30 minutes to 1 hour before meals, and at bedtime. Bedtime dose can be larger, and should be given at least 2 hours after last daily meal.
• Don't give an antacid at the same time as this drug because the antacid may interfere with drug absorption.
• Instruct patient to avoid driving or performing hazardous activities if he is drowsy, dizzy, or has blurred vision; to drink plenty of fluids to help prevent constipation; and to report any skin rash. Gum or sugarless hard candy may relieve mouth dryness.

• May aggravate symptoms of hyperthyroidism, coronary heart disease, congestive heart failure, cardiac arrhythmias, tachycardia, hypertension, or prostatic hypertrophy
• Takes effect rapidly, peaks at 3 to 4 hours, and lasts 6 to 10 hours
• Warn patient that drug may impair alertness or vision.
• Since oxybutynin suppresses perspiration, its use during very hot weather may precipitate fever or heat stroke.
• Store in tightly closed container at 60° to 85° F. (15° to 30° C).

We'd like to thank the following people and companies for their help with this PHOTOBOOK.

AMERICAN HEYER-SCHULTE CORP.
Goleta, Calif.

AMERICAN MEDICAL SYSTEMS INC.
Product Manager
Minneapolis, Minn.

C.R. BARD, INC.
Bard Urological Division
Murray Hill, N.J.

DACOMED CORPORATION
Minneapolis, Minn.
Paul C. Probst,
Director of Sales and Marketing

DAVOL INC.
Subsidiary of C.R. Bard, Inc.
Cranston, R.I.

EXTRACORPOREAL, INC.
King of Prussia, Pa.
Steven Hinkhouse,
Product Director

MEDICAL ENGINEERING CORP.
Racine, Wis.

NU-HOPE LABORATORIES, INC.
Los Angeles, Calif.
Eugene Galindo, President

NUMEDCO, INC.
Bridgeport, Pa.

PROCTER & GAMBLE CO.
Patient Care Products Division
Cincinnati, Ohio

RUSCH INC.
New York, N.Y.

SWEEN CORPORATION
Lake Crystal, Minn.
M. A. Sween, President

TRAVENOL LABORATORIES, INC.
Deerfield, Ill.

John Anderson, MD
William Gadbois, MD
Department of Urology
St. Luke's Hospital
Bethlehem, Pa.

Arthur Bogert, DO
Rolling Hill Hospital
Elkins Park, Pa.

George H. Snyder, III
Treasurer, Second Alarmers Rescue Squad
Willow Grove, Pa.

Also the staff of:

ALBERT EINSTEIN MEDICAL CENTER
Northern Division
Philadelphia, Pa.

Selected references

Books

ASSESSING YOUR PATIENTS. Nursing Photobook™ Series. Springhouse, Pa.: Intermed Communications, Inc., 1980.

Boyarski, Saul. TOTAL CARE OF THE PATIENT WITH A NEUROGENIC BLADDER. Boston: Little, Brown & Co., 1979.

Brundage, Dorothy J. NURSING MANAGEMENT OF RENAL PROBLEMS. St. Louis: C.V. Mosby Co., 1976.

Brunner, Lillian S. LIPPINCOTT MANUAL OF NURSING PRACTICE, 2nd ed. New York: J.B. Lippincott Co., 1978.

Brunner, Lillian S., et al. TEXTBOOK OF MEDICAL-SURGICAL NURSING, 4th ed. New York: J.B. Lippincott Co., 1980.

Cameron, Stewart J., et al. NEPHROLOGY FOR NURSES—A MODERN APPROACH TO THE KIDNEY. Garden City, N.Y.: Medical Examination Publishing Co., Inc., 1977.

Chaffee, Ellen E., and Esther M. Greisheimer. BASIC PHYSIOLOGY AND ANATOMY, 3rd ed. New York: J.B. Lippincott Co., 1974.

Chatterjee, Satya N., ed. RENAL TRANSPLANTATION. New York: Raven Press, Pubs., 1980.

DEALING WITH EMERGENCIES. Nursing Photobook™ Series. Springhouse, Pa.: Intermed Communications, Inc., 1980.

Geschickter, Charles F., and Tatiana T. Antonovych. KIDNEY IN HEALTH AND DISEASE. New York: J.B. Lippincott Co., 1971.

Gutch, C.F., and Martha H. Stoner. REVIEW OF HEMODIALYSIS FOR NURSES AND DIALYSIS PERSONNEL. St. Louis: C.V. Mosby Co., 1975.

Hansen, Ginny L., et al. CARING FOR PATIENTS WITH CHRONIC RENAL DISEASE. New York: J.B. Lippincott Co., 1974.

Harrison, J. Hartwell, et al. CAMPBELL'S UROLOGY, vol. 3, 4th ed. Philadelphia: W.B. Saunders Co.,1979.

Hole, John W., Jr. HUMAN ANATOMY AND PHYSIOLOGY. Dubuque, Iowa: Wm. C. Brown Co., 1978.

Kuehnelian, John G., and Virginia E. Sanders. UROLOGIC NURSING. New York: Macmillan Publishing Co., Inc., 1970.

Kunin, Calvin M. DETECTION, PREVENTION, AND MANAGEMENT OF URINARY TRACT INFECTIONS: A MANUAL FOR THE PHYSICIAN, NURSE, AND ALLIED HEALTH WORKER, 3rd ed. Philadelphia: Lea & Febiger, 1979.

Maude, David L. KIDNEY PHYSIOLOGY AND KIDNEY DISEASE: AN INTRODUCTION TO NEPHROLOGY. New York: J.B. Lippincott Co., 1977.

Morel, Alice, and Gilbert J. Wise. UROLOGIC ENDOSCOPIC PROCEDURES. St. Louis: C.V. Mosby Co., 1974.

Netter, Frank H., illus. THE CIBA COLLECTION OF MEDICAL ILLUSTRATIONS, vol. 6, *Kidneys, Ureters, and Urinary Bladder.* Summit, N.J.: CIBA Pharmaceutical Co., 1974.

Papper, Solomon. CLINICAL NEPHROLOGY, 2nd ed. Boston: Little, Brown & Co., 1978.

PERFORMING GI PROCEDURES. Nursing Photobook™ Series. Springhouse, Pa.: Intermed Communications, Inc., 1981.

Roen, Philip R. ATLAS OF UROLOGIC SURGERY. New York: Appleton-Century-Crofts, 1967.

Sachs, Bonnie L. RENAL TRANSPLANTATION—A NURSING PERSPECTIVE. Garden City, N.Y.: Medical Examination Publishing Co., Inc., 1977.

Smith, Donald R. GENERAL UROLOGY, 9th ed. Los Altos, Calif.: Lange Medical Publications, 1978.

Smith, Dorothy, and Carol P. Germain. CARE OF THE ADULT PATIENT. New York: J.B. Lippincott Co., 1975.

Tucker, Susan, and Mary Anne Breeding. PATIENT CARE STANDARDS. St. Louis: C.V. Mosby Co., 1975.

Winter, C. Chester., and Alice Morel. NURSING CARE OF PATIENTS WITH UROLOGIC DISEASES. St. Louis: C.V. Mosby Co., 1977.

Periodicals

Barrett, Nancy. *Continent Vesicostomy: The Dry Urinary Diversion*, AMERICAN JOURNAL OF NURSING. 79:462-464, March 1979.

DeGroot, Jane. *Catheter-Induced Urinary Tract Infections: How We Can Prevent Them*, NURSING76. 6:34-37, August 1976.

DeGroot, Jane. *Urethral Catheterization*, NURSING76. 6: 51-55, December 1976.

Hartman, Martha. *Intermittent Self-Catheterization*, NURSING78. 8:72-75, November 1978.

Juliani, Louise, and Bonita Reamer. *Kidney Transplant: Your Role in Aftercare*, NURSING77. 7:46-53, October 1977.

Kobrzycki, Paula. *Renal Transplant Complications*. AMERICAN JOURNAL OF NURSING. 77:641, April 1977.

McGuckin, Maryanne B. *Getting Better Urine Specimens with the Clean-Catch Technique*, NURSING81. 11:72-3, January 1981.

Sophie, Laura R. *Meeting the Immunologic Challenge of Transplant Nursing*, HEART & LUNG. 9:690-694, July-August 1980.

Stamm, Walter E. *Guidelines for Prevention of Catheter-Associated Urinary Tract Infections*, ANNALS OF INTERNAL MEDICINE. 82:386-390, March 1975.

Stillman, Margot. *Pre- and Postop Care of a Kidney Transplant Patient: What You Need to Know*, RN. 42:55-63, April 1979.

Selected references for the patient with a urologic problem

Chyatte, Samuel B. ON BORROWED TIME: LIVING WITH HEMODIALYSIS. Oradell, N.J.: Medical Economics Co., 1979.

Coleman, John W. SO YOU'RE GOING TO HAVE A CYSTOSCOPY. Norwich, N.Y.: Norwich-Eaton Pharmaceuticals, 1980.

Daut, R.V. SO YOU'RE GOING TO HAVE A PROSTATECTOMY. Norwich, New York: Eaton Laboratories, 1974.

Jeter, Katherine F. URINARY OSTOMIES—A GUIDEBOOK FOR PATIENTS. Los Angeles: United Ostomy Association, Inc., 1978.

MANAGING A UROSTOMY. Chicago: Hollister Inc., 1974.

Sugar, Elayne C. YOUR CHILD & REFLUX SURGERY: URETERAL REIMPLANT. Norwich, New York: Norwich-Eaton Pharmaceuticals, 1980.

WHAT EVERYONE SHOULD KNOW ABOUT KIDNEYS AND KIDNEY DISEASES. Greenfield, Mass.: Channing L. Bete Co., Inc., 1979.

Available from the Department of Health, Education, and Welfare, Washington, DC 20203:
KIDNEY DISEASE AND ARTIFICIAL KIDNEYS. Publication No. 74-376.
LIVING WITH END STAGE RENAL DISEASE. Publication No. 76-3001.

Index

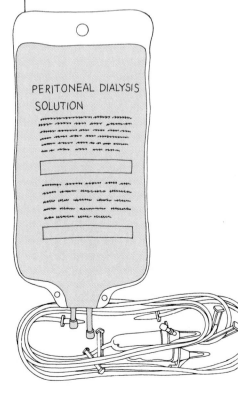

Index